Preface

The dietary survey of British schoolchildren was commissioned by the then Department of Health and Social Security and the Scottish Home and Health Department in response to the recommendation of the Committee on Medical Aspects of Food Policy's Sub-committee on Nutritional Surveillance that the effect of the new arrangements for school meals following the Education Act, 1980[1] should be monitored. As such it is part of their long term programme to monitor the effects of aspects of national food policy.

Fieldwork was completed in 1983 and a preliminary report of a nutritional analysis of this survey published in 1986[2] gave a description of the methods and the sampling used in the survey and the results of the analyses of the dietary patterns, the energy and nutrient intakes and the heights and weights of different groups of children in Great Britain. The Preliminary Report did not contain details of the survey carried out on an enhanced sample of primary schoolchildren in Scotland, nor analyses of the consumption of individual foods by different groups of children, nor information on how food and nutrient intake were distributed within the population. Only national average consumption of a limited number of groups of food was available, so it was not possible to explain the nutritional findings in terms of the individual foods consumed by any group. The quality and balance of the diets of children could not be assessed other than in terms of intakes of nutrients.

Analyses of the data to cover these matters have now been completed and a report on the diets of British schoolchildren in 1983 is presented which gives an account of the methods and findings for Great Britain as a whole and, where applicable, for Scotland.

Thanks are due to members of the Sub-committee on Nutritional Surveillance and its Working Group on School Meals, and to Mr I Knight and Mr J Eldridge of the Social Survey Division of the Office of Population Censuses and Surveys which carried out the fieldwork and processing of the data.

Sir Donald Acheson
Chairman of Committee on Medical Aspects of Food Policy

Contents

Summary

1. Statistical analysis and interpretation

1.1 This Report deals with the dietary habits of British schoolchildren and the contribution made by school meals in 1983. Since then many Local Education Authorities have introduced active policies to encourage healthy eating, accompanied in the last 4 years by health promotion campaigns, in the light of the publication of the COMA Report on Diet and Cardiovascular Disease in 1984[3], and other reports on diet and health[4].

1.2 Data are presented on the food and nutrient intakes of a representative sample of British schoolchildren measured by a 7-day record. Most food and some nutrient intakes were not normally distributed and median values are given in the tables of results. Interpretation and commentary are restricted to findings which achieved statistical significance (p<0.05) by parametric analyses. No non-parametric statistical analyses were attempted but data are given in detail in the tables and for those wishing to examine them further, the computer database of the survey is also available through the National Data Archive. Full documentation of the database may be obtained from the Social Survey Division of the Office of Population Censuses and Surveys, (OPCS) London.

2. Foods consumed

2.1 The main sources of dietary energy in the diets of British schoolchildren were bread, chips, milk, biscuits, meat products, cake and puddings. Almost all children in the survey recorded consumption of chips, crisps, cakes and biscuits. Boys recorded more chips consumed than girls along with more milk, breakfast cereals and baked beans; girls recorded more fruit consumed and more girls drank fruit juice than boys. Yogurt, fizzy drinks and sweets were more popular among younger children. Older children recorded consumption of more tea and coffee (para 9.2).

2.2 Scottish primary school children appeared to have a distinctive dietary pattern. They recorded higher median consumption of beef, soups, milk, cheese, sausages, chocolates and sweets and lower median consumption of

ix

cakes, biscuits, puddings, potatoes, and in particular, of vegetables of all kinds than children in the other regions of Great Britain (paras 9.3.2, 9.4.2, 9.5.2, 9.6.2).

2.3   Chips and milk were the two major items of the diets which varied most with social class and other socio-economic variables. Higher median chip consumption was recorded among social classes IV and V (para 9.3.3, 9.4.3, 9.5.3, 9.6.3), children with unemployed fathers, children from families receiving Supplementary Benefit (paras 9.3.5, 9.4.5, 9.5.5, 9.6.5), children taking school meals and those older children who ate out of school at cafes etc (para 8.4.2). Conversely median milk consumption was lower among most of these groups.

3.   Heights and Weights

3.1   Nearly all groups of children were on average above the fiftieth centile of standards for both height and weight standards (para 6.5). They also had average Body Mass Indices (BMI) above those calculated from the fiftieth standard centiles (para 6.6).

3.2   Among the younger children, those from families with fathers who were unemployed were significantly shorter than those from families in social classes I, II and III non manual. Younger girls with fathers unemployed were also significantly shorter than those in social class IV (paras 7.3.1.1, 7.3.2.1).

3.3   The younger children and older boys from families in receipt of supplementary benefit were significantly shorter than those from families not receiving benefits (paras 7.5.1.1, 7.5.2.1, 7.5.3.1).

3.4   At least 5 per cent of girls aged 14/15 years were dieting to lose weight (para 6.3).

4.   Nutrient intakes

4.1   Differences between energy and nutrient intakes of groups of children reflected the median consumption of chips and milk (paras 6.8, 6.11, 7.2.3, 7.2.4, 7.3.1.4, 7.3.2.3, 7.3.3.2, 7.3.4.2, 7.5.1.3, 7.5.3.3, 7.5.4.2, 8.3.4.1, 8.4.2).

4.2   Average energy intakes were about 90 per cent of the existing Recommended Daily Amounts (RDA). There was no evidence to suggest that these intakes were inadequate (para 6.2).

4.3   The average proportion of energy from fat ranged from 37.4 to 38.7 per cent across the different age and sex groups, and three quarters of children had intakes of fat over the level of 35 per cent of their enegy recommended by the COMA Panel on Diet and Cardiovascular Disease. Milk and chips were the two major contributors to these fat intakes (para 6.11).

4.4 Nutrient intakes were compared with the Recommended Daily Amounts (RDA) set by COMA in 1979. These RDA are estimated so that the requirements of almost all members of a group of healthy people are met. In practice if the average intake of a nutrient is at or above the RDA it can be assumed that the requirements of almost all individuals have been met. While in any group there may be individuals with nutrient intakes below the RDA, this does not necessarily imply dietary deficiency, which can be established only by clinical and biochemical tests of nutritional status. COMA have recognised that the RDA for the UK need revision and the Panel on RDA is currently reviewing them (para 6.1).

4.5 Average and median nutrient intakes were above the RDA in all age and sex groups for protein, thiamin, nicotinic aicid equivalent and vitamin C (paras 6.9, 6.15, 6.17, 6.18).

4.6 Both mean and median iron intakes of girls were below the RDA. The clinical significance of these iron intakes is not clear without further studies of iron status (para 6.14).

4.7 Both the mean and median intakes of riboflavin of the older girls were below the RDA. These girls obtained less of their riboflavin from milk and breakfast cereals which are major sources of this vitamin (para 6.16).

4.8 Nearly 60 per cent of older girls had calcium intakes below the RDA. These girls consumed less milk, bread and other cereals which are the main dietary sources of calcium (para 6.13).

4.9 Scottish primary schoolchildren had lower average intakes of vitamin C, ß-carotene and retinol equivalent than children in the Great Britain sample, reflecting lower consumption of carrots and vegetables (paras 6.18, 6.20, 6.21).

5. School Meals and the Diet

5.1 Dietary patterns of foods consumed were to some extent dependent on the provision from school meals. Older children obtained over half the chips that they ate in the survey week from school meals, both free and paid for. Younger children obtained over half the buns and pastries they ate from these sources (para 8.4.2). However the total average daily intakes of energy and nutrients did not vary with the kind of meal eaten at weekday lunchtimes (paras 8.3.1, 8.3.2, 8.3.3, 8.3.4).

5.2 There were no significant differences between the average energy or nutrient intakes of children taking school meals from outlets offering a free choice cafeteria style service and those obtaining a fixed price—fixed menu school meal (para 8.6). When school meals were eaten they contributed on average between 30 and 43 per cent of average daily energy intakes (para 8.4.5).

5.3   Older children, especially girls, who ate out of school at places such as cafes, take-away or 'fast food' outlets chose meals which were low in many nutrients, particularly iron (paras 8.4.6, 8.4.7). Their average daily nutrient intakes were not made up to the levels of intake of the rest of the population by the meals they consumed at other times during the week. The overall nutritional quality of their diets was the poorest of any group surveyed (para 8.3.4.2).

5.4   The school meal was an important contributor of food energy to the diets of older children (para 8.4.5).

Committee on Medical Aspects of Food Policy Sub-committee on Nutritional Surveillance

Chairman

Professor J S Garrow

Department of Human Nutrition
Medical College of
St Bartholomew's and
the London Hospitals,
London

Members

Dr S Bingham (from 1988)

Dunn Clinical Nutrition Unit,
Cambridge

Dr D Coggon (from 1988)

MRC Environmental
Epidemiology Unit,
Southampton

Professor J V G A Durnin

Institute of Physiology,
University of Glasgow,
Glasgow

Dr P C Elwood (until 1987)

MRC Epidemiology Unit,
Cardiff

Professor H Goldstein (until 1983)

Department of Statistics
and Computing,
Institute of Education,
University of London,
London

Professor W W Holland

Department of Community
Medicine,
United Medical and Dental
Schools of Guy's and
St Thomas' Hospitals,
St Thomas' Campus,
London

Professor W P T James
(from 1988)

The Rowett Research Institute,
Aberdeen

Professor R D G Milner

Department of Paediatrics,
University of Sheffield,
Sheffield

Professor T E Oppé (until 1988)

Department of Paediatrics,
St Mary's Hospital Medical
School,
London

Professor P R Payne (from 1983)

Department of Human Nutrition,
London School of Hygiene
and Tropical Medicine,
London

Professor J M Tanner (until 1987)

Department of Growth and
Development,
Institute of Child Health,
University of London,
London

Professor J C Waterlow
(until 1983)

Department of Human Nutrition,
London School of Hygiene and
Tropical Medicine,
London

Dr R G Whitehead (until 1987)

Dunn Nutritional Laboratory,
Milton Road,
Cambridge

Assessors

Dr D H Buss

Ministry of Agriculture,
Fisheries and Food,
London

Dr M Hennigan

Scottish Home and Health
Department,
Edinburgh

Secretariat

Dr R K Skinner (medical)
(until 1986)

Department of Health,
London

Dr M J Wiseman (medical)
(from 1986)

Department of Health,
London

Mr R W Wenlock (scientific)
(from 1984)

Department of Health,
London

Mr K L G Follin (administrative)

Department of Health,
London

Committee on Medical Aspects of Food Policy
Sub-committee on Nutritional Surveillance
Working Group on School Meals

Chairman

Professor J S Garrow   Department of Human Nutrition
                                    Medical College of
                                    St Barthomolew's and
                                    the London Hospitals,
                                    London

Members

Professor J Durnin   Institute of Physiology,
                                    University of Glasgow,
                                    Glasgow

Dr P Elwood   MRC Epidemiology Unit,
                                    Cardiff

Professor W Holland   Department of Community
                                    Medicine,
                                    United Medical and Dental
                                    Schools of Guy's and
                                    St Thomas' Hospitals,
                                    London

Miss J Marr   Royal Free Hospital,
                                    London

Mr D Miller   Late of Queen Elizabeth College
                                    (now King's College)
                                    London

In attendance

Miss S Chinn   Department of Community
                                    Medicine,
                                    United Medical and Dental
                                    Schools of Guy's and
                                    St Thomas' Hospitals,
                                    London

Dr R Rona	Department of Community Medicine, United Medical and Dental Schools of Guy's and St Thomas' Hospitals, London

Observers

Mr T Ball	Department of Education and Science, London
Mr H Barrick	Department of Education and Science, London
Mr J Eldridge	Office of Population Censuses and Surveys, London
Mr I Knight	Office of Population Censuses and Surveys, London
Ms J Todd	Office of Population Censuses and Surveys, London
Dr J Ablett	Department of Health and Social Security, London
Miss P Bailey	Department of Health and Social Security, London
Dr S Fine	Department of Health and Social Security, London
Mrs E Lohani	Department of Health and Social Security, London
Dr S Rosenbaum	Department of Health and Social Security, London
Dr A Yarrow	Department of Health and Social Security, London

Secretariat

Dr R Skinner (medical)	Department of Health and Social Security, London
Mrs M Disselduff (scientific) (until 1984)	Department of Health and Social Security, London
Mr R Wenlock (scientific) (from 1984)	Department of Health and Social Security, London
Mr D Smith (administrative) (until 1982)	Department of Health and Social Security, London
Mr K Follin (administrative) (from 1982)	Department of Health and Social Security, London
Mrs N McAfee (minutes)	Department of Health and Social Security, London

1. Introduction

1.1 Prior to 1980 the meals provided by schools in England and Wales had to conform to prescribed nutritional standards. The 1980 Education Act[1] released Local Authorities from this requirement and left them free to decide the form, content and price of schools meals. Although Scotland had no nutritional standards for school meals prescribed by central Government, there was a regulation requiring that school meals be suitable and adequate in all respects as the main meal of the day for recipients. The 1980 Education (Scotland) Act revoked the earlier regulations and left Education Authorities free to decide the form and content of school meals. In the debate on these Acts, Ministers agreed to monitor the effect of the new arrangements. As a result the matter was referred to the Sub-committee on Nutritional Surveillance of the Committee on Medical Aspects of Food Policy (COMA) who recommended that a seven-day weighed measurement of food intake together with a study of the heights and weights of a nationally representative sample of schoolchildren should be carried out.

1.2 A Working Group on School Meals was set up by the Sub-committee to help plan and supervise this study. They proposed a survey which was commissioned with the Office of Population Censuses and Surveys (OPCS) by the Department of Health and Social Security (DHSS) and the Scottish Home and Health Department (SHHD) as part of their long term programme of monitoring the effects of many aspects of national food policy. In particular it was designed to examine the contribution of school meals to the overall diet of British schoolchildren.

1.3 This type of nutritional survey involves intensive fieldwork and each age group needs separate analysis. This made it impractical to cover all ages within the school population. Therefore two age groups of children aged 10 or 14 years at the start of the school year were selected. These were chosen in the hope that most of the younger girls would be pre menarchal and most of the older boys would have entered their adolescent growth spurt. The two age groups were thereby comparable with those selected in some previous DHSS dietary studies.[5] The Scottish Home and Health Department commissioned

1

an enhanced sample of children aged 10 years in Scotland in order to provide more representative data on their diets.

1.4   This Report deals with the dietary habits of schoolchildren and the contribution made by school meals in 1983. The fieldwork was carried out by OPCS on a sample of children aged 10/11 and 14/15 years between January and June 1983. Since 1983, many Local Education Authorities have introduced active policies to encourage healthy eating, accompanied by promotion campaigns, in the light of the publication of the COMA Report on Diet and Cardiovascular Disease[3] in 1984, and other reports on diet and health[4].

1.5   The selected children were all from Local Authority maintained schools in which school meals were provided, and the sample does not reflect the circumstances of children in, for example, independent schools or special schools.

1.6   A brief description of the sample and methodology is given below. A detailed description of the sample is given in Appendix A, the way in which the dietary records were collected is described in Appendix B, details of the anthropometric methods are given in Appendix C and examples of the fieldwork questionnaires, diaries and record books are given in Appendix D.

2. Survey Methodology

2.1 The survey sample in England and Wales

2.1.1 Sampling in England and Wales was based on a multi-stage design to select areas, then eligible schools, and finally children in the specified age groups. The first stage was a sample of Local Authority districts selected randomly with probability proportional to size of school population aged 11 to 15 years. Within the selected districts each secondary school was clustered with nearby primary schools and a sample of these clusters was then selected, again with probability proportional to the school population aged 11 to 15 years.

2.1.2 If this school population were spread between schools in the same proportions as the two age groups of interest, sampling theory would require an equal number of children to be selected from each school cluster. Also, the arrangements for the fieldwork required approximately equal numbers in each cluster. Inevitably the two age groups of interest were not distributed in exactly the same way as the school population aged 11 to 15 years and it was necessary to weight the sample at the processing stage to compensate for the unequal probabilities of selection.

2.1.3 In anticipation that children "at risk" of poor nutrition would be more likely to be found in the less advantaged families these children were oversampled to provide larger numbers for separate analysis. When reporting results for the national sample these groups were combined with the rest by weighting back to comprise only their true proportionate share of the total sample. However, for examining these special interest groups separately, their enhanced samples were available.

2.1.4 Although roughly equal numbers in the two age groups were planned, a larger sample of the secondary school age group resulted because response rates in the early stages of the survey, which started mainly in the secondary schools, were higher than expected. The school sample was reduced by random methods in order to contain the total cost of the survey.

2.2 The survey sample in Scotland

2.2.1 Sampling in Scotland was done differently. Primary and secondary schools were sampled independently. Secondary schools were selected with probability proportionate to the school population aged 11 to 15 years with a

3

constant number of children randomly selected from each school. Primary schools were grouped into contiguous clusters and the clusters were sampled according to the number of 10 year old children expected from the previous year's school census.

2.2.2   The primary schoolchildren were oversampled deliberately to allow a separate Scottish analysis, but within this report where a nationally representative British sample of younger children is discussed all Scottish results have been weighted to their proportionate share of the total sample. The data from the entire Scottish sample are also given where appropriate under the headings "Total Scotland Sample" and "Scottish 10/11 years". The sample of Scottish primary schoolchildren was also weighted to compensate for oversampling of children from the less advantaged families and unequal probabilities of selection for children from different school clusters, but this weighting was arranged so that the weighted total sample size equated to the number of completed interviews.

2.3   Response and non-response in Great Britain

2.3.1   The response levels for the combined Great Britain sample are described in detail in Appendix A. A small number of schools refused to co-operate which resulted in a loss of about 4 per cent of the eligible children. Some 7.5 per cent of the parents or children were unwilling to co-operate and a further 5.5 per cent dropped out during the record keeping week. On inspection of the completed record books the consultant nutritionists rejected another 4.5 per cent because of poor or dubious record keeping, while 3 per cent of children were not in the final sample for other reasons (eg non-contacts).

2.3.2   The final response rate was just over 75 per cent. A total of 3,296 successful 7 day records was achieved (see Appendix A) though not all of those had both heights and weights measured, so when the sample was weighted as described above, the composition of the final weighted Great Britain sample was:

	7-day dietary record	Heights measured	Weights measured
Boys aged 10/11 years	902	898	891
Girls aged 10/11 years	821	814	807
Boys aged 14/15 years	513	511	509
Girls aged 14/15 years	461	455	454
Totals	2,697	2,678	2,661

2.4   Response and non-response in Scotland

2.4.1   The response levels for the enhanced sample of Scottish primary schoolchildren are also described in Appendix A. Among the sampled

4

children eligible for a full interview, 4 per cent of the parents or the children themselves were unwilling to co-operate and a further 5.5 per cent dropped out during the record keeping week. On inspection of the completed record books the consultant nutritionists rejected a further 4.5 per cent for poor or dubious record keeping while 2.5 per cent of children were not in the sample for other reasons (eg non-contacts).

2.4.2   The final response rate in Scotland was just over 75 per cent. The composition of the final sample of Scottish primary schoolchildren was as follows:

	7-day dietary record	Heights measured	Weights measured
Boys aged 10/11 years	457	457	457
Girls aged 10/11 years	427	424	421
Totals	884	881	878

2.5   Dietary measurements

2.5.1   The fieldwork in this survey used methodology proposed by the Working Group on School Meals and developed by Mrs M M Disselduff of the DHSS Nutrition Unit.

2.5.2   The parents of all the selected children were first contacted by letter and given a chance to withdraw their children from the survey. Thereafter an OPCS fieldworker made direct contact and held an interview in which questions were asked about the child's eating habits and family situation, and the nature of the survey was then explained in more detail.

2.5.3   The children and their parents were told how everything the child ate and drank should be recorded for the next 7 days. They were taught how to weigh on digital scales and to record in considerable detail the child's food and any leftovers. The fieldworker returned within 24 hours to check that the records were being kept with sufficient detail and accuracy, and to probe for further information on entries recorded with inadequate detail. Children were given pocket notebooks to record any food or drink consumed away from home where weighing was not possible, and fieldworkers were usually able to trace the sources of that food and buy and weigh a duplicate. For those taking school meals special arrangements were made to have complementary record books and scales available in the school canteens.

2.5.4   Checking calls were made on each child during the recording week and some children who were not very good at recording were visited daily. In general, the children co-operated in the survey with great enthusiasm.

2.6 Anthropometric measurements

2.6.1   As the children were to be surveyed at ages when there was a potential for rapid growth, the Working Group on School Meals advised that heights and weights should be measured. The methods developed by OPCS in their Survey of Adult Heights and Weights[6] were used (Appendix C). Height was measured with the OPCS portable stadiometer, calibrated in mm. Weight was measured using a SOEHNLE personal weighing scale with a digital readout calibrated in 200g units.

2.6.2   Heavy outer garments were removed, but no specific allowance has been made for weight of clothing in this Report.

3. Sample Structure

3.1 **Socio-economic status** The Department of Employment's Family Expenditure Survey shows that family expenditure on food varies with socio-economic status. For families where the head of the household is employed, social class based on occupation is an indicator of socio-economic position. However in families where the father is unemployed social class is not useful. In Table 1 children are grouped under headings which described their father's current employment status, ie long-term sick or disabled, unemployed and "other" which included children whose fathers were retired, students or otherwise out of the labour market. One parent families are also shown separately.

3.2 **Employment and unemployment** Table 1 shows that 11 per cent of the children sampled had a father who was unemployed, including one per cent whose fathers were laid off as sick and expecting to find a job when well. In addition around 2 per cent had a father who was long-term sick or disabled. Of the Scottish primary schoolchildren 13 per cent had a father who was unemployed and 2.5 per cent had a father who was long-term sick or disabled. There were too few children with long-term sick fathers to be analysed separately, and they have been aggregated with the unemployed group. The 1.5 per cent of children in the 'other' category have not been included in subsequent analyses.

3.3 **Family composition** Table 2 shows that a marginally greater proportion of children in the older age group came from one parent families than in the younger age group. The younger children were more likely than the older ones to come from families with other dependent children, because more siblings of the older group were likely to have grown beyond the age of dependence.

3.4 **Regional breakdown** The sample was not large enough for a detailed regional breakdown but Table 3 shows the distribution between Scotland (the weighted Scotland sample for 10/11 year olds), the North (including Northern, North Western and Yorkshire/Humberside regions), London and the South East, and the rest of Britain. The numbers in Wales were too small to produce reliable separate estimates.

3.5 **Social Security Benefits** Table 4 shows that 2.5 per cent of children in all age groups came from families receiving Family Income Supplement (FIS). In the younger age group 16.5 per cent were from families receiving Supplementary Benefit (SB) as were 14.0 per cent of the older children. A small proportion (0.5 per cent) came from families that received both FIS and SB in the survey week. In Scotland the corresponding figures for primary schoolchildren were 3.5 per cent from families receiving FIS and 16.5 per cent from families receiving SB.

3.6 **School meals** There are many variations in the way schoolchildren receive and consume meals at lunchtime. For instance school meals can be free or paid for, be served on a cafeteria or on a fixed price system fixed menu basis. The Working Group on School Meals advised that for children of all ages the type of lunchtime meal should be analysed in the following groups:

    Paid school meals daily (Paid)
    Free school meal daily (Free)
    Paid school meal most days (Paid most days)
    Free school meal most days (Free most days)
    Meal at home all or most days (Home)
    Packed lunch all or most days (Packed lunch)

In addition, an extra group "cafe or take away meal all or most days" (Cafe) was included, though too few younger children ate out of school in this way for meaningful separate analysis. The two basic school meal systems—the cafeteria type offering a choice of foods to the children and the fixed price which presents a menu offering little or no choice—were analysed separately. Those schools offering a hybrid of these two systems or a packed lunch only to those in receipt of free school meals have been classified as 'other' and analyses are reported where sufficient children were surveyed.

3.7 **Ethnic origin** The survey included children of different ethnic origins, in proportion to their numbers in each age group in the schools. Although there were local concentrations of children from different ethnic groups, the Working Group on School Meals advised that the total numbers from the minority ethnic groups were too small for valid separate analysis. The foods commonly consumed by populations immigrant to Britain[7] were included in the nutrient data base constructed for this survey (see para 4.1).

4. Dietary Analysis

4.1 The nutrient database

4.1.1 All foods consumed by each child during the survey week were recorded and allocated a code from a specially constructed nutrient database which had been prepared by the Nutrition Branch of the Food Science Division of the Ministry of Agriculture, Fisheries and Food (MAFF). The 1,080 different food items were those for which estimates of the nutrient composition were available in 1982. To supplement the tables of food composition[8], new analyses were included for bread and cereal products[9], immigrant foods[7] and some cooked dishes[10]. The recipe dishes from the DHSS Food Composition Tables were recalculated using these recent data. This means that the nutrient database used in this survey is not strictly comparable with previous DHSS studies on similar age groups carried out between 1968 and 1971[5]. The nutrient database was constructed to allow intakes to be calculated for the following:

Energy	Nicotinic acid
Fat	Nicotinic acid equivalent
Carbohydrate (as monosaccharides)	Retinol
Protein	Carotene
Calcium	Retinol equivalent
Iron	Vitamin D
Thiamin	Pyridoxine (Vitamin B6)
Riboflavin	

The nutrient database was constructed in 1982 when computer facilities for use in calculating recipes were limited and there were problems with values for many minor nutrients. Therefore individual fatty acids (for which insufficient data was available to allocate values for cooked dishes), sucrose and other sugars, and dietary fibre are excluded.

4.1.2 Item coding in nutritional studies of this type may result in the aggregation of foods which vary in their composition. For example, 'deep fried potato chips' included all home-prepared and cooked chips (excluding those purchased frozen which were recorded separately). Chips eaten outside the home obtained from school canteens, fish and chip shops and franchised 'fast food' outlets are known to vary in nutrient content, particularly fat. A check on the most recent analyses of chips was carried out (MAFF unpublished). The values from the British tables of food composition[8] were found still to be representative for these products and were used for all deep fried potato chips recorded in the survey.

4.2 **The scope of dietary analysis** The Preliminary Report of this survey[1] provided an analysis of children's heights, weights and energy and nutrient intakes. Only national averages of foods consumed were available for 38 groups of foodstuffs which had been aggregated for convenience. For this Report full descriptions of the diets of different sub-groups including Scotland and the English regions have now been prepared. These are given for 75 individual foods and groups of foods in tables 34 to 57. In these tables the potatoes eaten are divided into crisps (which includes similar snack-type foods) chips, (which includes all chips as discussed in para 4.1.2) and potatoes (which includes all other potatoes including mashed, boiled, roast and potato salad).

5. Statistical Analysis and Interpretation

5.1 **The survey database** This Report provides data on heights, weights and food and nutrient intakes. These were available from a computerised database compiled from the documents and records of the survey (see Appendix D). This database is available from the National Data Archive at the University of Essex, Colchester. The documentation describing the production and format of the database is also available from the Social Survey Division of the Office of Population Censuses and Surveys, London.

5.2 **Statistical analysis** Interpretation and commentary have been restricted to findings which are normally distributed and were significant ($p<0.05$). Most food and some nutrient intakes were not normally distributed and nearly half of the distributions were still skewed after logarithimic transformation. Parametric statistical tests were therefore not appropriate and have not been done. The data are given in as much detail as possible in the tables and are available in the computerised database for those wishing to examine any relationships in more detail.

5.3 **Means and medians** Intakes of food and some nutrients were not normally distributed because there were always children who consumed none of certain foods in the survey week or only a little of the more popular foods. Distributions were therefore positively skewed and though mean (average) intakes were calculated in each case, their value for interpretation was limited. Therefore medians, ie the values of the middle observations when all the observations were listed in order from the lowest to the highest, were also calculated. As the median divides a distribution into halves, it is a more useful index where there is a high degree of skew. The calculation of medians on weighted data is explained in detail in para 6, Appendix A.

5.4 **The reporting of nutrient intakes** Although the distributions of food consumption were skewed, the distributions of most daily energy and nutrient intakes were not skewed, probably due to the variety of food consumption. Therefore daily energy and nutrient intakes are given as arithemtic means with standard deviations. Medians are also given in figures and tables and where nutrient intakes were not normally distributed this is stated. Differences in energy intake were tested for significance parametrically and are reported in the text.

11

6. Heights, Weights and the Energy and Nutrient Intakes

6.1 Recommended intakes, nutrient requirements and growth standards

6.1.1   The nutrient intakes of the children were compared with the existing DHSS recommended daily amounts (RDA) of nutrients[11]. These RDA, which are under review by the Committee on Medical Aspects of Food policy, were estimated so that requirements of almost all members of a group of healthy people are met. Consequently they are higher than average nutrient *requirements*. In practice if the *mean* (average) intake of a nutrient is at or above the RDA it can be assumed that the requirements of almost all individuals have been met. While in any group there may be individuals with nutrient intakes below the RDA, this does not necessarily imply dietary deficiency, which can be established only by clinical and biochemical tests of nutritional status.

6.1.2   The RDA for dietary energy in contrast to those of nutrients, is based on estimated *mean* requirements of populations who are neither losing nor gaining weight, (or, in the case of children, growing at a normal rate); therefore half the individuals in any group should have energy intakes below the RDA.

6.1.3   Children who receive sufficient energy and nutrients to meet their individual requirements should grow adequately. Growth is assessed by comparing heights and weights with appropriate reference standards. In Britain the data of Tanner, Whitehouse and Takaishi published in 1966[12] are those most commonly used. These "Tanner standards" were based on measurements of normal British children made in 1959 and they were adjusted in 1965. The Sub-committee on Nutritional Surveillance recommended that they be used in this study as the best available. They are referred to as 'standards' throughout this Report.

6.2   **Energy intakes**   The average daily energy intake of the 14/15 year old boys was higher than those of the younger boys (p.<0.01) and the average intakes of energy by boys were higher than those of the girls in both age groups (p.<0.01, table 5, Fig 6.1). Separate analyses of heights, weights and intakes of most nutrients and of energy showed no statistically significant differences between Scottish primary school children and the 10/11 year olds

12

in the Great Britain sample. Mean energy intakes were about 10 per cent lower than the existing RDA, a finding common to recent British surveys of food intakes. Mean weights and heights were calculated for each of the ranges of energy intake given in table 5 (tables 6 and 7). The children were, on average, on or above the fiftieth centile of standards for height and well above the fiftieth centile of standards for weight, regardless of energy intake.

6.3 **Slimming** There was no coded question for slimming diets on the survey forms but interviewers noted that 22 of the older girls (5 per cent) claimed to be dieting to lose weight. This was in line with recent findings from a nationwide sample of teenagers studied at about the same time where 6 per cent of girls aged 15–18 years said they were on a diet to lose weight[13]. Dieting complicates the interpretation of both food consumption and nutrient intakes by the older girls. Thirteen of the 67 girls with energy intakes up to 6MJ per day claimed to be dieting to lose weight. The intakes of other nutrients by these girls were therefore also likely to be reduced by dieting.

6.4 **Pubertal growth spurts** The wide range of heights and large standard deviations in Table 6 are probably due to variation in the age of the pubertal growth spurt. Some girls approaching their eleventh birthday may have already entered puberty and be growing rapidly. Most girls have completed their growth in height by their fifteenth birthday. Very few boys start their growth spurt by their eleventh birthday. However the growth rate among most boys is at a maximum in their fifteenth year.

6.5 **Weights and energy intakes** The data in Table 7 do not show low weight for age for any group of children. On average weights were above the fiftieth centile of the standards. The 67 girls aged 14/15 years with the lowest recorded average energy intakes (up to 6MJ per day) were also those with the highest average weights.

6.6 **Body Mass Index** Body Mass Index (BMI) is a crude measure of the fatness of an individual and is calculated as $\dfrac{wt(kg)}{ht(m)^2}$.

BMI was calculated for each child for whom both height and weight measurements were available and the means are shown compared with values calculated from the fiftieth centiles of standard heights and weights as follows:

Age/sex group	n	BMI mean	s.d	Fiftieth standard centile
Boys 10/11 years	898	17.9	3.1	16.4
Girls 10/11 years	805	18.0	3.0	17.0
Boys 14/15 years	509	19.9	2.6	19.3
Girls 14/15 years	452	20.7	3.2	20.3

On average children of each age and sex, particularly the younger children, were heavier for their heights than the appropriate fiftieth standard centile. However the children were weighed with light clothing while those weighed to produce the standards were weighed in underclothes only,[12] and this may have contributed to differences in BMI. Further analyses showed that there was no significant difference between the sexes at either age and there was no significant correlation between BMI and energy intake for either age or sex (tables 6 and 7). However the 67 older girls with energy intakes of less than 6 MJ per day had a mean BMI of 23.8 (sd 4.8) compared with the overall mean of 20.7(sd 3.2). Thirteen of these girls claimed to be dieting to lose weight. BMI was not found to be correlated with socio-economic category.

6.7   **Contribution of foods to nutrient intakes**   In the discussions that follow the distribution of intakes of each nutrient by the Great Britain and Scottish samples is given as a histogram along with the arithmetic mean, its standard deviation, the median and, where appropriate, the RDA[11]. The intakes of nutrients by Scottish primary schoolchildren were so similar to those of the Great Britain samples of 10/11 year olds that they are discussed separately only where a major difference was found. The patterns of food intakes are given in tables 34 to 57. To help interpret nutrient intakes, all foods found to contribute 5 per cent or more to the intakes of energy or each nutrient are listed for the Great Britain sample in table 8. Similar lists for Scotland are given in Table 9.

6.8   **Energy**   The distribution of energy intakes is given in figure 6.1. The main individual sources of energy in the diets of British school children were bread, chips, milk, biscuits, meat products, cakes and puddings, which together accounted for about half the energy intake (Table 8).

6.9   **Protein**   The distribution of protein intakes is given in figure 6.2. The RDA for protein is calculated as 10 per cent of the energy RDA. Mean intakes of energy from protein were as follows:

Protein as per cent of energy intakes

	Mean	sd	n
Boys aged 10/11 years	12.0	1.6	902
Girls aged 10/11 years	11.8	1.7	821
Boys aged 14/15 years	12.3	1.7	513
Girls aged 14/15 years	12.4	2.2	461

6.10   **Fat**   The distribution of fat intakes is given in figure 6.3. About half of the fat in the diets of the children was obtained from milk, chips, meat products, biscuits, carcase meats, crisps and butter (table 8) The food making the single greatest contribution to fat intakes in the younger children was milk (12 per cent of fat intake) and that in older children was chips (11 per cent of fat intake).

14

6.11 **Fat as a percentage of energy intakes**   There is no existing RDA set for fat but the proportion of energy derived from fat is considered to be important in relation to the development of cardiovascular and other diseases[2]. Distributions of fat intake as percentage of energy provided by fat are given in figure 6.4. Mean and median contributions of fat to energy were as follows:

Fat as per cent of energy intakes

	Median	Mean	sd	number
Boys aged 10/11 years	37.6	37.4	3.3	902
Girls aged 10/11 years	38.1	37.9	3.5	821
Boys aged 14/15 years	37.8	37.9	3.7	513
Girls aged 14/15 years	38.6	38.7	3.7	461

Approximately one quarter to one third of children had fat intakes contributing more than 40 per cent of their energy intakes and three quarters took more than 35 per cent of their energy as fat (fig. 6.4). This contrasts with the recommendation of the COMA Panel on Diet and Cardiovascular Disease[2] that total fat intake should not exceed 35 per cent of energy. Unfortunately, insufficient data on the fatty acid composition of cooked food and recipe dishes were available to allow separate analyses of fatty acid intakes. On average younger children derived 4 per cent of their energy from fat in milk they drank and the older children about 3.5 per cent. Older boys and girls also derived 3 and 4 per cent respectively of their energy from fat in chips (Table 8).

6.12 **Carbohydrate**   The distribution of carbohydrate intakes (expressed as monosaccharides) is given in figure 6.5. Carbohydrate was the main source of energy for all children. On average the proportion of energy derived from carbohydrate was as follows:

Carbohydrate as per cent of energy intakes

	Mean	sd	number
Boys aged 10/11 years	50.5	3.8	902
Girls aged 10/11 years	50.2	4.0	821
Boys aged 14/15 years	49.8	4.1	513
Girls aged 14/15 years	48.8	4.3	461

6.13 **Calcium**   The distribution of calcium intakes is given in figure 6.6. The boys had mean intakes well above the RDA. However older girls had a mean intake which was lower than the RDA for 15 year olds, and 57 per cent consumed less than 700mg per day. The main source of calcium for all children was liquid milk which contributed on average between 30 and 37 per cent. Other major sources were bread, cheese and puddings (Table 8).

15

6.14 **Iron** The distribution of iron intakes is given in figure 6.7. Mean intakes of all children, except older boys, were below the RDA. Normally about 10 per cent of dietary iron is absorbed[11] but in deficiency the efficiency of iron absorption increases[14]. Some older girls on very low intakes, for instance those on slimming diets, are at high risk of iron deficiency, particularly if they have heavy menstrual losses[15]. The main sources of iron were bread and breakfast cereals and, to a lesser extent chips, carcase meats and other meat products (table 8).

6.15 **Thiamin** The distribution of thiamin intakes is given in figure 6.8. Average intakes in all groups were above the RDA. The main dietary sources of thiamin were breakfast cereals, which provided on average between 16 and 27 per cent, and bread, carcase meats, milk, chips and potatoes (Table 8).

6.16 **Riboflavin** The distribution of riboflavin intakes is given in figure 6.9. All groups, except the older girls, had mean intakes above the RDA. Nearly 60 per cent of the older girls consumed less than 1.4mg per day. Milk and breakfast cereals were the major sources of riboflavin for all children but older girls derived less riboflavin from these foods (Table 8). Riboflavin deficiency is not seen in Great Britain and without further biochemical data it is difficult to assess whether these dietary findings have any clinical significance.

6.17 **Nicotinic acid equivalent** The vitamin nicotinic acid is available preformed from foods and is also produced in the body from the amino acid tryptophan. Figure 6.10 shows total intakes as the nicotinic acid equivalent available from both sources. All groups had mean intakes well above the RDA.

6.18 **Vitamin C** Both mean and median intakes were well above the RDA in all groups (fig 6.11). Among the older boys in Great Britain chips provided 25 per cent of vitamin C intakes (table 8). Children also obtained vitamin C from vegetables, potatoes, fruit and fruit juices. The Scottish primary school children had lower median vitamin C intakes. The main differences in their diets appeared to be a contribution to vitamin C intakes from vegetables of only 9 to 13 per cent (table 9) compared with 15 to 19 per cent for the Great Britain sample (table 8) and the contribution from chips was 19 to 32 per cent (table 9) compared with 16 to 20 per cent for the Great Britain sample (table 8).

6.19 **Retinol** the distribution of retinol intakes is given in figure 6.12. Preformed retinol is present in fortified margarines and in foods of animal origin, particularly liver, but also in milk, milk products, eggs and butter. The distribution was positively skewed, and girls had lower median intakes.

6.20 **ß Carotene** The distributions of ß carotene intakes given in figure 6.13 were also positively skewed. This nutrient occurs mainly in vegetable foods, particularly carrots, and the very wide distributions probably reflect large variations in the consumption of carrots and other vegetables. The Scottish primary schoolchildren had lower median intakes.

6.21 **Retinol equivalent** About 6 µg ß carotene is converted to 1 µg retinol in the body. The total available retinol is thus preformed retinol plus that derived from ß carotene and is expressed as retinol equivalent. The distributions of intakes given in figure 6.14 were very skewed and median intakes were below the RDA. Carrots and liver are such rich sources of retinol equivalent that distributions were skewed by those children consuming larger quantities of carrots or any liver during the survey week. However, on average, liver consumption contributed less than 5 per cent of the retinol equivalent intakes of any age of sex group. The main sources of this vitamin were carrots, milk, butter, vegetables, cheese and margarine (table 8). The median intakes of Scottish primary schoolchildren were lower than those of the 10/11 year olds in the Great Britain sample. Milk and cheese were the major sources of retinol equivalent for Scottish primary schoolchildren (table 9). They derived 9 to 16 per cent of their retinol equivalent from carrots and between 5 and 7 per cent from soups which could contain carrots. They derived less than 5 per cent from vegetables compared with 6 to 8 per cent for children in Great Britain (table 8).

6.22 **Vitamin D** Vitamin D intakes were skewed (Fig 6.15). This nutrient is found only in foods of animal origin, particularly liver, fatty fish and eggs, in margarine and in breakfast cereals fortified with vitamin D. The chief source of vitamin D is not the diet but synthesis in the body following the action of ultra-violet light on the skin. No RDA was therefore set[11], except for children aged less than 5 years, and for women during pregnancy and lactation. However, some adolescents may need 10 µg vitamin D per day as a supplement during a period of rapid skeletal growth, especially during the winter months when exposure to sunlight may be inadequate for their needs which are unlikely to be met by the diet. Fortified margarines provided on average 22 to 27 per cent of vitamin D intakes, with eggs and breakfast cereals being the other main sources (table 8).

6.23 **Pyridoxine (vitamin B6)** The distributions of intakes of pyridoxine (vitamin B6) are given in figure 6.16. There is no existing RDA set in the UK for this nutrient[11], but the National Academy of Sciences of the USA has set a Recommended Dietary Allowance for children aged 11 to 14 years of 1.8 mg per day[16]. Mean intakes were below this but there is no evidence of pyridoxine deficiency in Britain. Potatoes were the main sources of this nutrient. Potatoes, crisps and chips together provided between 31 and 35 per cent of the intake of pyridoxine with milk, carcase meats and bread the other major sources (table 8).

7. Energy and Nutrient Intakes and Socio-economic Variables

7.1 **Introduction** The energy and nutrient intakes of the different groups of children are given in tables 10 to 21 according to region, social class, family composition, employment and benefit status. The means and standard deviations of the heights of the children in each of these divisions are also provided.

7.2 **Region** The heights and energy and nutrient intakes of 10/11 year old and 14/15 year old children are given in tables 10 and 11 respectively. There were no significant differences between the heights of any group of children of either age and sex from the different regions, including Scotland.

7.2.1 *Boys aged 10/11 years* The mean energy intake of Scottish boys was lower than that of boys from the North and those from London and the South East but these differences were not statistically significant. However, the nutrient intakes did show some regional patterns. Scottish boys consumed on average the least fat, retinol, carotene, retinol equivalent, vitamin D, pyridoxine, and, in particular, vitamin C (table 10). The contributions of various foods to these nutrient intakes are given in table 9, particularly the lower contributions of carrots and vegetables to Scottish intakes of retinol equivalent. In contrast, boys from London and the South East had the highest intakes of fat, carbohydrate and vitamin C, the last reflecting the popularity among these boys of fruit juices, which provided 24 per cent of the intake.

7.2.2. *Girls aged 10/11 years* Mean energy intakes of younger girls were similar across the regions, but the pattern of nutrient intakes varied (table 10). Scottish girls had the lowest intakes of retinol, carotene, retinol equivalent, thiamin, riboflavin, nicotinic acid equivalent, vitamin D and pyridoxine. In particular, like the boys, they had the lowest vitamin C intakes—72 per cent of the intakes of girls from London and the South East. The higher vitamin C intakes of girls from London and the South East reflected the popularity of fresh vegetables and fruit juices which provided 16 and 23 per cent respectively of the vitamin C.

7.2.3 *Boys aged 14/15 years* The differences between the regional mean energy intakes of the older boys were not statistically significant (table 11).

18

Scottish boys obtained 12 per cent of their fat and 32 per cent of their vitamin C from chips as did those from the North. Boys from London and the South East obtained 7 per cent of their fat and 19 per cent of their vitamin C from chips. Scottish boys derived 26 per cent of their vitamin D from margarine while those from London and the South East derived 20 per cent.

7.2.4 *Girls aged 14/15 years* There were no statistically significant differences between regional energy intakes. However the pattern of nutrient intakes, with lower vitamin C, retinol, carotene, retinol equivalent, vitamin D and iron intakes among Scottish girls (table 11), was as in the other age and sex groups and reflected the Scottish dietary pattern shown in table 9. Older girls from London and the South East had the highest vitamin C intakes. Vegetables and fruit juices were popular; they obtained 15 per cent of their vitamin C from chips while girls from Scotland and the North obtained 22 and 23 per cent respectively from this source. They derived 20 per cent of their vitamin D intakes from margarine while Scottish girls derived 31 per cent.

7.3 **Social class and height** The OPCS survey of Adult Heights and Weights[6] showed that in Great Britain height of normal adults is related to social class, with younger men aged 16 to 19 years in social classes I and II being 3.5cm (2.0 per cent) taller on average than those in social classes IV and V. For women this difference is 3.4cm (2.1 per cent)[6]. Social class differences in height are established by age 2½ years[17] and the National Study of Health and Growth has shown that this social class difference in heights persists among primary school children aged 5 to 11 years[18,19]. The reason for these differences is not fully understood but it is speculated that there may be a nutritional component[6]. A relationship between height and social class was therefore expected for children in this survey. The mean heights and energy and nutrient intakes of children in families with a father are given in tables 12 to 15 by social class and employment status. Because of small numbers of children in social classes I and V, for statistical analyses social classes I and II, and IV and V were combined and published in the Preliminary Report of the Survey[2], but the full data are now presented in tables 12 to 15 with social classes disaggregated.

7.3.1 *Boys aged 10/11 years*

7.3.1.1 The mean heights given in table 12 show the expected trend with social class. The children of fathers who were unemployed or long term sick were significantly shorter than those in social classes I and II (p<0.001) and those in social class IIInm (p<0.01), but not significantly shorter than social classes IIIm, IV and V. In 1983 unemployment was commonest among social classes IIIm, IV and V[6] and the heights of younger boys from families with unemployed fathers may have reflected this social class difference. No allowance was made for parental heights.

7.3.1.2 The energy intakes of the younger boys in social classes I and II were significantly higher (p<0.05) than those in classes IV and V[2]. There was a tendency for energy intake to decline with social class but those in class IIInm had unexpectedly lower energy intakes (p<0.01) than those in class IIIm as well as those in classes I and II (p<0.01)[2]. This may have been due to the inclusion of a concentration of boys of Asian origin in the sample of social class IIInm (see para 9.3.3.)

7.3.1.3 The boys from families where the father was unemployed had energy intakes which were the same as those from social classes I and II and significantly higher that those in classes IIInm (p<0.01) and classes IV and V (p<0.05)[2].

7.3.1.4 Although there were no significant differences in their patterns of nutrient intakes, the mean vitamin C intake of the boys from social class I was 12.4mg per day higher than that of boys from social class V. Among the former, 27 per cent of vitamin C intake was derived from fruit juice, 17 per cent from vegetables and less than 15 per cent from chips, while social class V derived 21 per cent from chips and less than 15 per cent from either of the other two sources. The mean calcium intake of boys from social class I was also higher by 120mg per day that that of boys from social class V. Milk was a major contributor of calcium, thiamin, riboflavin, nicotinic acid equivalent, retinol equivalent and pyridoxine (table 8) and differences in milk consumption were reflected in the fall with social class of mean intakes of these nutrients. Again, the nutrient intakes of boys from social class IIInm did not fit in with these trends (see para 9.9.3).

7.3.1.5 The intakes of nutrients by boys from families where the father was unemployed were generally similar to those from families of social classes IV and V.

7.3.2 *Girls aged 10/11 years*

7.2.3.1 None of the differences in height between social classes was statistically significant (table 13). However the girls from families where the father was unemployed were significantly shorter than girls from each of the social classes I to IV (p<0.05 in all cases).

7.3.2.2 The energy intakes among the younger girls given in table 13 showed no consistent relationship with social class or employment status.

7.3.2.3 Mean intakes of some nutrients tended to fall with social class. Girls from families with a father unemployed had nutrient intakes similar to those of social classes IV and V. As with the younger boys the sources of nutrients varied. The contributions of nutrients from milk fell with social class and with unemployment while those from chips rose, as shown in the following tables.

Per cent of nutrients from milk

Girls aged 10/11 years

Social Class	Energy	Fat	Fat as per cent of energy	Calcium	Pyridoxine
National average	7	12	4	32	8
I	9	13	5	39	10
II	8	11	4	34	9
IIInm	8	11	4	33	9
IIIm	7	10	4	33	8
IV	6	8	3	30	7
V	6	8	3	27	7
unemployed	6	8	3	28	7

Per cent of nutrients from chips

Girls aged 10/11 years

	Energy	Fat	Fat as per cent of energy	Iron	Vitamin C	Thiamin
National average	8	8	4	6	16	6
I	5	5	2	4	8	3
II	6	6	2	4	10	4
IIInm	8	8	3	6	13	5
IIIm	8	8	3	6	17	6
IV	9	9	3	7	19	7
V	11	11	4	8	23	9
unemployed	11	11	4	8	23	8

Younger girls from social class V or with unemployed fathers obtained over twice as much of their fat, vitamin C, iron and thiamin from chips and those from social class I, while obtaining only about 75 per cent as much fat, calcium and pyridoxine from milk.

7.3.3 *Boys aged 14/15 years*

7.3.3.1   There was a tendency for the older boys from social classes IV and V to be shorter than those from other social classes but the differences were not statistically significant (table 14).

7.3.3.2 There were no statistically significant differences between the energy intakes of the older boys. There were data from only 11 boys from social class V. These are given in brackets as they were too few for valid separate statistical analyses. Fat, iron, thiamin and vitamin C intakes all fell with social class. However, these falls are associated in each case with a rise in the proportion of intake derived from chips as follows:

Per cent of nutrients from chips

Boys aged 14/15 years

Social Class	Energy	Fat	Fat as per cent of energy	Iron	Thiamin	Vitamin C
National average	11	11	4	8	8	25
I	7	7	3	5	5	17
II	10	10	4	8	7	19
IIInm	10	10	4	7	7	22
IIIm	10	10	4	8	7	23
IV	12	12	4	9	8	29
V	14	14	5	10	10	29
Unemployed	14	15	6	11	11	36

Older boys with fathers unemployed obtained 15 per cent of their energy from the fat in the chips they ate. They also obtained more of their iron, thiamin and, particularly, vitamin C from chips than boys from any of the social classes.

7.3.4 *Girls aged 14/15 years*

7.3.4.1 There were no statistically significant differences between the heights of the older girls (table 15).

7.3.4.2 The differences between energy intakes among social classes were not statistically significant. Girls from social class I had the highest intakes of iron, retinol equivalent, thiamin, riboflavin, nicotinic acid equivalent and vitamin C and pyridoxine. Thirty per cent of their vitamin C intake was derived from vegetables, 20 per cent from fruit juice and only 20 per cent from chips. Girls who were reported to be dieting were evenly distributed between social classes. There were too few older girls from social class V for separate analysis but those from class IV had the lowest intakes of fat, calcium, iron, retinol equivalent, thiamin, riboflavin and vitamin D. Lower consumption of milk could account for most of these differences; only 28 per cent of their calcium intake was from this source.

7.3.4.3   The girls from families where the father was unemployed were not significantly shorter than those from families with a father in employment. Their pattern of nutrient intakes did not differ from those with a father in employment. Girls who were reported to be dieting were evenly distributed between families with a father unemployed or in employment.

7.4   **Family composition**   The energy and nutrient intakes of children from one and two parent families are given in tables 16 to 19 according to the number of children in the family. One parent households might be considered as a vulnerable group and some differences between one and two parent families for heights and intakes and energy and nutrients might be expected. Height is known to be related to family size, as defined by the number of children, those with more siblings tending to be shorter[20].

7.4.1   *Heights*   When the heights of children from two and one parent families were compared, there were no significant differences for any age and sex. There was a relationship between height and the number of siblings in two parent families. Children from families with four or more children were the shortest in all age and sex groups but none of the differences was statistically significant.

7.4.2   No consistent relationship of family size or number of parents with the energy and nutrient intakes of any group of children was found.

7.5   **Supplementary Benefit and Family Income Supplement**   The heights and energy and nutrient intakes of children from families whose fathers were unemployed or on low incomes are given in tables 20 and 21.

7.5.1   *Boys aged 10/11 years*

7.5.1.1   Younger boys from families not receiving benefits were 2.9cm taller than those from families receiving SB ($p < 0.001$).

7.5.1.2   There were no significant differences in energy intake between younger boys from families in receipt of FIS, SB or not in receipt of benefits.

7.5.1.3   None of the differences in nutrient intakes between children from families in receipt of benefit and those from families not receiving benefits were statistically significant. The only major dietary difference was the high proportion of nutrient intakes derived from chips by boys from families receiving SB with 11 per cent of their fat and 24 per cent of their vitamin C intakes derived from this source compared with the national averages of 8 and 16 per cent respectively (table 8).

7.5.2 *Girls aged 10/11 years*

7.5.2.1 Younger girls from families receiving SB were 2.7cm shorter (p<0.05) than those not receiving benefits.

7.5.2.2 There were no significant differences in energy and nutrient intakes between younger girls from families in receipt of FIS, SB or not in receipt of benefits.

7.5.3 *Boys aged 14/15 years*

7.5.3.1 Older boys from families receiving SB were 2.9cm shorter (p<0.05) than those from families not receiving benefits.

7.5.3.2 There were no significant differences in energy intakes between older boys from families in receipt of FIS, SB or not in receipt of benefits.

7.5.3.3 Intakes of nutrients reflected energy intakes with boys from families on SB showing only slightly lower intakes of all nutrients, particularly vitamin C. Chips were a major source of nutrients for these older boys (table 8), especially for those from families receiving SB as shown below.

Per cent of nutrients derived from chips

Boys aged 14/15 years

Nutrient	FIS	SB	Neither FIS or SB	National average
Energy	13	15	11	11
Fat	13	15	11	11
Fat as per cent of energy	5	6	4	4
Iron	10	11	8	8
Thiamin	10	11	8	8
Vitamin C	33	37	23	25

Older boys from families in receipt of SB obtained 15 per cent of their fat and 37 per cent of their vitamin C from chips. This corresponds closely with the data for older boys from families with the father unemployed given in para 7.3.3.2 where 15 and 36 per cent respectively of fat and vitamin C were derived from chips.

7.5.4 *Girls aged 14/15 years*

7.5.4.1 There was no significant difference between the heights of children from families receiving SB and those from families not receiving benefits.

7.5.4.2   There were no significant differences in energy or nutrient intakes between older girls from families in receipt of FIS, SB or not in receipt of benefits. Girls who claimed to be dieting were evenly distributed in each group. Older girls from families receiving SB derived 14 per cent of their fat and 27 per cent of their vitamin C intakes from chips compared with national average figures of 11 and 20 per cent respectively.

8. School Meals and Nutrient Intakes

8.1 **The Education Act, 1980** Before 1980, the school meals provided by Local Education Authorities in England and Wales had to meet prescribed nutritional standards—ie one third of the appropriate Recommended Daily Intake (RDI)[21] for energy and 40 per cent of that for protein. Local Education Authorities in Scotland were expected to ensure that the school meals be suitable in all respects as the main meal of the day for recipients. These requirements were not retained in the 1980 Acts and the RDI used in the legislation were superseded by the 1979 RDA[11] which were lower. The Sub-committee on Nutritional Surveillance advised that in 1983, when the survey was carried out, it would be reasonable to expect a school meal to provide about one third of the children's actual daily energy intake. To examine this, the contributions of lunchtime food to the average daily energy and nutrient intakes have been calculated for different subgroups of children according to their weekday lunchtime meal arrangements.

8.2 **Classification of weekday lunchtime meals** For the analysis reported here the weekday lunchtime meal has been classified in the following groups:

Paid school meal daily (Paid)
Free school meal daily (Free)
Paid school meal most days (Paid most days)
Free school meal most days (Free most days)
Meal at home all or most days (Home)
Packed lunch all or most days (Packed lunch)
Cafe or take away meal all or most days (Cafe)

8.3 **Daily nutrient intake according to weekday lunchtime meal** The mean heights and energy and nutrient intakes of British schoolchildren analysed according to weekday lunchtime meal are given in tables 22 to 25. Nutrient intakes have been calculated from all foods consumed during the seven days of the survey, including weekends.

8.3.1 *Boys aged 10/11 years*

8.3.1.1 Younger boys taking free school meals every day were significantly shorter (p<0.01) than those taking paid school meals every day (Table 22).

Those taking free school meals most days were significantly shorter (p<0.05) than those paying for their school meal most days.

8.3.1.2   There were no significant differences between the energy intakes of boys on any lunchtime meal regime. Those taking free school meals had the lowest daily intakes of vitamin C, of which they obtained 26 per cent from chips.

8.3.1.3   *Scotland*   Separate analyses of the Scottish primary school sample showed no significant differences for heights, energy or nutrient intakes between the boys in Scotland and those of the Great Britain sample.

8.3.2   *Girls aged 10/11 years*

8.3.2.1   Those girls who took free school meals daily were significantly shorter than those who paid for their school meal every day (p<0.05), those who took free school meals most days (p<0.05) and those who took packed lunches (p<0.001) (Table 23).

8.3.2.2   There were no significant differences between the daily energy intakes of any of the younger girls.

8.3.2.3   *Scotland*   As with the younger boys, the Scottish primary school girls showed no significant differences between their heights, energy and nutrient intakes and those of the Great Britain sample.

8.3.3   *Boys aged 14/15 years*

8.3.3.1   There were no significant differences between the heights of any of the groups of older boys (Table 24).

8.3.3.2   There were no significant differences between the energy intakes of these boys, and the patterns of intakes of all nutrients were very similar regardless of the type of lunch consumed.

8.3.4   *Girls aged 14/15 years*

8.3.4.1   There were no significant differences between the heights of these girls (Table 25). However, the girls who went home for lunch consumed 1,150kJ per day less than those who received a free school meal every day (p<0.01). Those taking free school meals derived 17 per cent of both their energy and fat from chips. These were the highest proportions from chips of any group of children of either age and sex studied in the survey. They also derived 35 per cent of their vitamin C intake from chips. Girls who claimed to be dieting were evenly distributed among these groups.

8.3.4.2 Of the older girls, 54 (11 per cent) ate out of school at cafes etc at lunchtime. Although their daily energy intakes were no different from other groups of older girls, they had the lowest intakes of iron, and of protein, calcium, carotene, retinol equivalent, nicotinic acid equivalent and vitamin D. The nutritional quality of the daily diets of these girls, in terms of nutrients per MJ, was lower than in any other group of older girls taking lunch from any other source.

8.4 Weekday lunchtime nutrient intakes from school meals and other sources

8.4.1 During the survey the children recorded all food consumed at weekday lunch times and food eaten as a school meal was recorded separately from all other food eaten. Some schools have tuck shops and children also took sweets, chocolates, and other items to eat with a school meal. These were recorded separately, but if they were consumed at lunchtime they were included as part of the lunchtime food intake.

8.4.2 Chips, buns and pastries dominated the weekday lunches of school-children. The percentage of the mean weekly consumption of these was as follows:

Per cent of mean weekday consumption obtained at lunchtime of chips, buns and pastries according to type of meal

	Chips			Buns and pastries		
Age/sex Group	Paid school meal	Free school meal	Cafe	Paid school meal	Free school meal	Cafe
Boys 10/11 years	41	35	—	57	52	—
Girls 10/11 years	39	34	—	52	54	—
Boys 14/15 years	58	51	52	45	60	14
Girls 14/15 years	58	58	44	37	32	58

Older children obtained over 50 per cent of their daily weekday consumption of chips from school meals. For younger children the school meal was the major daily source of buns and pastries. Older girls who ate out at cafes etc obtained the majority of these foods then.

8.4.3 In order to assess the contribution of the food eaten at weekday lunchtimes to the daily diets of the children surveyed, the energy and nutrients obtained during weekday lunchtimes have been averaged over five days, excluding the weekend, and are given in tables 26 to 29. The adequacy of the meal for each group has been estimated as the percentage of the children's average total daily energy intake over the same five day period.

The percentage of energy derived from fat in the meal consumed at lunchtime is also shown.

8.4.4 The average proportion of energy from fat in the lunchtime meal eaten away from home varied between 39 and 45 per cent. For meals taken at home it was 38 to 40 per cent. Mean fat intakes were between 37 and 39 per cent of energy (see para 6.10) so other meals eaten at home must have been providing on average less than 37 per cent of their energy as fat.

8.4.5 When this survey was carried out in 1983 between 70 and 80 per cent of the children receiving free school meals came from families receiving benefits. The rest received free school meals under the discretion granted to Local Authorities. It was shown in Section 7 that the energy and nutrient intakes of children from families in receipt of benefits who may have qualified for free school meals, and those with unemployed fathers and from one parent families, were similar to those of other groups. The proportions of the daily intake of energy provided by the type of mid-day meal were as follows:

Age/sex group	Free school meal	Paid school meal	Home	Cafe
	(per cent of daily energy intake)			
Boys 10/11 years	31	30	31	28
Girls 10/11 years	31	30	30	33
Boys 14/15 years	39	36	32	33
Girls 14/15 years	43	39	32	32

The patterns for those taking school meals most days, both free or paid for, were similar except for the older boys who obtained 22 and 25 per cent of their daily energy intakes from school meals respectively. Older children depended more than younger children on the school meal for their daily energy intakes.

8.4.6 The proportion of daily energy intakes obtained by older children who ate out of school was similar to that of children who took a midday meal at home. However the nutritional quality of their lunchtime meals was lower. In particular, the older boys obtained the lowest amounts of protein, calcium, iron, retinol equivalent, thiamin, riboflavin and nicotinic acid equivalent from their cafe meals (table 28). The older girls also obtained the lowest amounts of protein, calcium, iron, retinol equivalent, thiamin, riboflavin, nicotinic acid equivalent and vitamin D from these sources (table 29).

8.4.7 These low nutrient intakes from a "cafe" meal appear to be compensated for by intakes from other meals by the boys during the week as

29

shown previously in table 24. However from table 25 it appears that the older girls only partly made up their intakes of iron in particular and protein, calcium, nicotinic acid equivalent and vitamin D from other meals.

8.5 Weekday lunch time nutrient intakes from school meals and other sources by Scottish primary schoolchildren The same analyses of the nutritional contribution of school meals were carried out on the total sample of Scottish primary schoolchildren and the results are given in tables 30 and 31. The patterns revealed were very similar to those for the younger children in the Great Britain sample given in tables 26 and 27.

8.6 Daily nutrient intake according to type of school meal

8.6.1 *Type of school meal* Children taking school meals received them from a cafeteria style outlet, a fixed price outlet with limited or no choice or from a school meal system which offered both or some other provision such as sandwiches. The patterns of nutrient consumption of children eating school meals from these outlets are given in tables 32 and 33.

8.6.2 There were no major differences between the patterns of energy or nutrient intakes between any of the children in any age and sex group obtaining school meals from the three types of outlet.

9. Dietary Patterns

9.1 **Presentation of food intakes** The median and arithmetic mean food intakes are given in tables 34 to 57. Where less than 50 per cent of the children consumed a food in the survey week, the median value was zero. In these cases the arithmetic mean consumption by those children who were recorded as eating the food is given in brackets and the number of such children is given immediately below.

9.2 **Age and sex difference** The daily energy intakes of boys and girls and of older and younger children have already been shown to be significantly different (para 6.2). All the children consumed large quantities of bread, cakes, biscuits, puddings, milk, meat products, crisps, potatoes and particularly large quantities of chips. The older boys had the highest median consumption of chips. The consumption of many foods varied with age and sex. Boys drank more milk, and ate more breakfast cereals, cheese, meat products, potatoes and baked beans than girls. Older children ate more chips, white bread and poultry and drank more tea than younger children while these in turn ate more puddings and drank more fizzy drinks. However, when further analysed by region, socio-economic status, lunchtime meal regime and type of school meal there were few major variations in the patterns of food consumption. Those which were apparent from tables 34 to 57 are discussed below with those features of the dietary patterns which accounted for the differences in the nutrient intakes described earlier in this Report.

9.3 Dietary patterns of boys aged 10/11 years

9.3.1 *Great Britain* The dietary patterns of the boys aged 10/11 years in the weighted Great Britain sample are given in tables 34 to 39. The national medians show a general pattern of consumption of large quantities of chips, bread, cakes, biscuits, breakfast cereals, milk, puddings and meat products along with nearly half a litre per week of fizzy drinks (table 34).

9.3.2 *Scotland* Compared with the medians for Great Britain in table 34 the younger boys from Scotland had lower median consumption of vegetables, cakes, biscuits, puddings, other meat products and potatoes and higher consumption of beef, milk, cheese, sausages, chocolate and sweets (Table 35). Soups were particularly popular among Scottish boys which reflects the finding in table 9 that soups provide 6 per cent of their retinol equivalent intakes, probably due to the carrots in the soups. This Scottish pattern is distinctive and reflects findings from the National Food Survey.[22]

9.3.3 *Social class* The consumption of chips tended to increase between social classes I and V, boys from social class V eating over twice as much chips as those from social class I. A similar trend was apparent for other meat products, sugar and sweets. There was an opposite trend for milk, chocolate and vegetables. Fruit juices were more popular among social classes I and II (table 34). The boys from social class IIInm did not conform to this social class pattern. This may have been due to the inclusion of a concentration of children of Asian origin in this sample from social class IIInm. These boys tended to follow traditional Asian dietary patterns of eating more rice, pasta, yogurt, butter and other fats and less bread, cakes, milk, cheese, pig meat, beef, sausages and chips than might otherwise have been expected.

9.3.4 *Family composition* The dietary patterns of younger boys were not related to family composition (table 36).

9.3.5 *Employment and benefits* Boys from families where the father was unemployed had dietary patterns very similar to those of boys from families where the father was in employment (table 37); however median chip consumption of boys from families with a father unemployed was 40 per cent higher. As was discussed earlier, boys from families receiving SB derived more of their average fat and vitamin C intakes from chips (see para 7.5.1.3). Their median consumption was 522 grams per week compared with 380 grams per week by boys from families not receiving benefits (table 37).

9.3.6 *Type of lunch* The type of lunch consumed during the school week did not influence dietary patterns. As expected, those taking a packed lunch had the highest consumption of bread, biscuits, margarine, cheese, crisps and apples. Otherwise those taking school meals, whether free or paid for, have very similar dietary patterns (table 38).

9.3.7 *Type of school meal* There were no major differences between the dietary patterns of the younger boys according to the three types of outlet that provided their school meals (table 39).

9.4 Dietary patterns of girls aged 10/11 years

9.4.1 The dietary patterns of the younger girls are shown in tables 40 to 45. The national medians (table 40) confirm the tendency for younger girls to consume less white bread and cereal products in general and milk, meat products, chips and potatoes than other age and sex groups.

9.4.2 *Scotland* The medians show that the primary school girls in Scotland (table 41) have the same distinctive dietary pattern as the younger boys.

Soups were often eaten and contributed 7 per cent of retinol equivalent intakes (table 9). They had lower median consumption of many vegetable and carrots were less popular than among the younger girls in the Great Britain sample. This also explains in part the contributions to vitamin C and retinol equivalent intakes given in table 9 and is typical of the Scottish household food purchase pattern shown by the National Food Survey.[22]

9.4.3 *Social class* The contribution of chips to the nutrient intakes of the younger girls rose between social classes I and V while the contribution from milk fell (see para 7.3.2.3). The girls from social class V ate nearly three times as much chips than those from social class class I, while median milk consumption by girls from social class V was only 68 per cent of the median for social class I (table 40).

9.4.4 *Family composition* The dietary patterns of younger girls were not related to family composition (table 42).

9.4.5 *Employment and benefits* It was shown previously that younger girls from families with the father unemployed obtained the smallest proportions of several nutrients from milk and the largest proportions from chips (see para 7.2.2.3). The median milk consumption of these girls was 1,106g per week compared with 1,403g per week for girls from families where the father was in employment (table 43). Those with unemployed fathers also ate nearly 50 per cent more chips. There were no major differences in the patterns of food consumption by the girls whether or not they came from families in receipt of benefits.

9.4.6 *Type of lunch* The type of lunch consumed during the school week did not markedly influence dietary patterns (table 44). Those taking a packed lunch ate more margarine, biscuits, yogurts, cheese, crisps and fruit and drank more fruit juices and soft drinks. Those going home for lunch ate the most chips and the least burgers and other meat products, biscuits, carrots, peas, other vegetables and colas and consumed the most milk, lamb and fizzy drinks. There were no major differences between those paying for or receiving free school meals, though the consumption of fruit juices by the latter was low.

9.4.7 *Type of school meal* There were no major differences between the dietary patterns of the younger girls according to the three types of outlet that provided their school meals (table 45).

9.5 Dietary patterns of boys aged 14/15 years

9.5.1 The dietary patterns of the older boys are shown in tables 46 to 51. There was a tendency for older boys to consume more than younger boys of most foods, but, in particular chips, bread and milk.

9.5.2 *Region*   The regional data are from the Great Britain sample (table 47). The Scottish dietary pattern shown previously by the younger children was also shown by the older boys. Those from Scotland and boys from the North had a median chip consumption 30 to 50 per cent higher than those of boys from the other English regions. Scottish boys drank more milk and ate more cheese. This is in line with National Food Survey data.[22]

9.5.3 *Social class*   Varying comsumption of chips was found previously to be the reason for the difference in the proportions of the nutrient intakes of these older boys (see para 7.3.3). The median consumption of chips doubled from 320 grams per week for social class I to 766 grams per week for social class V, while median milk consumption by boys from social class V was only half that of boys from social class I (Table 46).

9.5.4 *Family composition*   The dietary patterns of the older boys were not related to family composition (table 8).

9.5.5 *Employment and benefits*   The median chip consumption of boys from families with a father unemployed was 826 grams per week which was 40 per cent greater than the median consumption of those from families with a father in employment (Table 49). The median consumption of chips by older boys from families receiving SB was 917 grams per week, over 40 per cent greater than the median of boys from families not receiving benefits.

9.5.6 *Type of lunch*   The type of lunch consumed during the school week did not markedly influence dietary patterns (table 50). As with the younger children the older boys who took a packed lunch to school had the highest consumption of bread, biscuits, crisps, other vegetables and apples. There were 68 older boys who ate out of school at cafes, take-away and fast food outlets. These boys were eating a self-selected meal at week-day lunch times, and they ate the most eggs, other meat products, chocolate and colas.

9.5.7 *Type of school meal*   Only 4 older boys ate school meals from outlets in the 'other' category and the data for these are not shown (table 51). There were no differences between the dietary patterns of the older boys obtaining a school meal from either a cafeteria or fixed price outlet.

9.6   Dietary patterns of girls aged 14/15 years

9.6.1   The dietary patterns of the older girls are shown in tables 52 to 57. The older girls ate differently from both older boys and the younger girls. They consumed more food in general than younger girls, reflecting their greater energy requirements, but they had lower median consumption of cakes, biscuits, puddings, milk, sweets, crisps, baked beans, tea and fizzy drinks than the younger girls.

9.6.2 *Region* The distinctive Scottish dietary pattern is also apparent among the older girls from Scotland, who had the lowest median consumption of milk (table 53). Vegetables and fruit juices were less popular while beef and soups were more popular than among the girls from the English regions. Fruit juices were particularly popular among the girls from London and the South East.

9.6.3 *Social class* As described previously there were few differences in nutrient intakes with social class among the older girls, except for the proportions of nutrients derived from chips, milk and fruit juice (see para 7.3.4.2). Median chip consumption rose between social classes I and V and median milk consumption fell. Fruit juice consumption was particularly high among these older girls but its popularity fell between class I and class V (table 54).

9.6.4 *Family composition* The dietary patterns of the older girls were not related to family composition (table 54).

9.6.5 *Employment and benefits* The dietary data from the 10 girls from families in receipt of FIS are given for information only (table 55). None of the differences between the dietary patterns of older girls from families with fathers unemployed or in employment were large enough for separate comment. The girls from families with a father unemployed or receiving SB had the highest median consumption of chips.

9.6.6 *Type of lunch* The type of lunch consumed during the school week did not markedly influence dietary patterns (table 56). As with the rest of children those girls taking a packed lunch to school ate the most bread, biscuits, crisps and apples. There were 54 girls who ate out of school at cafes, take-away and fast food outlets. Like the older boys in this category they were eating a self-selected meal at week-day lunch times. They ate the most eggs, bacon, poultry, sausages, burgers, chocolate, other vegetables, colas and fizzy drinks. The nutritional significance of these choices has been discussed. (See paras 8.3.4.2 and 8.4.6).

9.6.7 *Type of school meal* There were no major differences between the dietary patterns of the older girls according to whether they obtained a school meal from either the cafeteria or fixed price system (table 57).

References

1 *Education Act 1980*. London: HMSO, 1980.

2 Wenlock RW, Disselduff MM, Skinner RK, Knight I. *The diets of British schoolchildren: preliminary report of a nutritional analysis of a nationwide dietary survey of British schoolchildren*. London: Department of Health and Social Security, 1986.

3 Panel on Diet in Relation to Cardiovascular Disease. *Diet and cardiovascular disease*. London: HMSO, 1984. Chairman: P.J. Randle. (Reports on health and social subjects; 28).

4 National Advisory Committee on Nutrition Education. *A discussion paper on proposals for nutritional guidelines for health education in Britain*. London: Health Education Council, 1983. Chairman: W P T James.

5 Darke SJ, Disselduff MM, Try GP. Frequency distributions of mean intakes of food, energy and selected nutrients obtained during nutrition surveys of different groups of people in Great Britain between 1968 and 1971. *Br J Nutr 1980*; **44**: 243–252.

6 Knight I, Eldridge J. *The heights and weights of adults in Great Britain: report of a survey carried out on behalf of the Department of Health and Social Security covering adults aged 16–64*. London: HMSO, 1984.

7 Tan SP, Wenlock RW, Buss DH. *Immigrant foods: second supplement to McCance and Widdowson's The Composition of Foods*. London: HMSO, 1985.

8 Paul AA, Southgate DAT. *McCance and Widdowson's The Composition of Foods*. 4th ed. London: HMSO, 1978.

9 Holland B, Unwin ID, Buss DH. *Cereals and cereal products: third supplement to McCance and Widdowson's The Composition of Foods*. Letchworth: Royal Society of Chemistry, 1988.

10 Wiles SJ, Nettleton PA, Black AA, Nutrient composition of some cooked dishes eaten in Britain: a supplementary food composition table. *Hum Nutr Appl Nutr 1983*; **34**: 189–223.

11 Department of Health and Social Security. *Recommended daily amounts of food energy and nutrients for groups of people in the United Kingdom*. London: HMSO, 1979. (Reports on health and social subjects; 15).

12 Tanner JM, Whitehouse RH, Takaishi M. Standards from birth to maturity for height, weight, height velocity and weight velocity: British children, 1965. *Arch Dis Child 1966*; **41**: 454–471, 613–635.

13 Bull NL. Dietary habits of 15-to-18 year-olds. *Hum Nutr Appl Nutr 1985;* **39A** (suppl 1): 1–68.

14 Monsen ER, Hallberg L, Layrisse M, et al. Estimation of available dietary iron. *Am J Clin Nutr 1978;* **31**: 134–141.

15 Barker SA, Bull NL, Buss DH. Low iron intakes among young women in Britain. *Br Med J [Clin Res] 1985;* **290**: 743–744.

16 Food and Nutrition Board Staff. *Recommended dietary allowances*. 9th ed. Washington DC: National Academic Press, 1980.

17 Department of Health and Social Security. *Second report of the Sub-committee on Nutritional Surveillance*. London: HMSO, 1981. Chairman: A M Thomson. (Report on health and social subjects; 21).

18 Rona RJ, Swann AV, Altman DG. Social factors and height of primary schoolchildren in England and Scotland. *J Epidemiol Community Health 1978*; **32:** 147–154.

19 Department of Health. *Third report of the Sub-committee on Nutritional Surveillance: executive summary*. London: HMSO, 1988. Chairman: J S Garrow. (Report on health and social subjects; 33).

20 Rona RJ, Florey CV. National study of health and growth: respiratory symptoms and height in primary schoolchildren. *Int J Epidemiol 1980;* **9**: 35–43.

21 Department of Health and Social Security. *Recommended intakes of nutrients for the United Kingdom*. London: HMSO, 1969. (Reports on public health and social subjects; 120).

22 Ministry of Agriculture, Fisheries and Food. *Food consumption and expenditure* 1986. London: HMSO, 1988.

List of Tables

Table 1: *Socio-economic status of families (per cent of children)*

	One parent families	Two parent families Social Class (father working)					Father not working		
		I	II	IIInm	IIIm	IV+V	Unem-ployed	Long-term Sick	Other
All 10/11 year olds	12	6	23	10	22	12	11	1.5	1.5
Scottish 10/11 year olds	14	5	18	9	23	14	13	2.5	1.5
14/15 year olds	16	6	17	8	22	15	11	2.5	1.5

Table 2: *Family composition (per cent of children)*

	10/11 year olds		Scottish 10/11 year olds		14/15 year olds	
	one parent	two parents	one parent	two parents	one parent	two parents
1 child	3.0	12.0	3.0	12.0	9.0	38.0
2 children	6.0	48.0	6.5	42.0	4.0	28.0
3 children	3.0	19.0	4.0	21.5	2.0	11.0
4 or more children	0.5	8.5	1.0	10.0	0.5	7.0
Total	12.5	87.5	14.5	85.5	15.5	84.0

Table 3: *Geographical distribution by age of schoolchildren in the Great Britain sample (per cent of children)*

	10/11 year olds	14/15 year olds
Scotland	9 (weighted)	10
North	31	28
London and South East	26	29
Rest of Britain	34	33

Table 4: *Families receiving family income supplement or supplementary benefit (per cent of children)*

	10/11 year olds	Scottish 10/11 year olds	14/15 year olds
Supplementary Benefit (SB)	16.5	16.5	14.0
Family Income Supplement (FIS)	2.5	3.5	2.5
Both SB and FIS	0.5	0.5	0.5
Neither	80.5	79.5	83.0

Table 5: *Daily intake of energy (kJ)*

Energy	Aged 10/11		Aged 14/15	
	Boys	Girls	Boys	Girls
kJ	%	%	%	%
4,000 – 5,000	0	3	0	5
5,001 – 6,000	2	7	1	10
6,001 – 7,000	9	22	4	15
7,001 – 8,000	22	32	10	24
8,001 – 9,000	27	20	13	21
9,001 –10,000	21	10	18	15
10,001–11,000	11	3	15	8
11,001–12,000	5	2	17	2
12,001–13,000	1	0	11	0
13,001–14,000	1	0	6	0
14,001–15,000	0	0	3	0
over 15,000	0	0	2	0
Average kJ(s.d)	8,670(1,510)	7,690(1,610)	10,400(2,300)	7,850(1,740)
kcal	2,070	1,840	2,480	1,870
Median kJ	8,610	7,570	10,230	7,880
RDA kJ	9,500	8,500	11,500	9,000
Number of children	902	821	513	461

Table 6: *Average heights[1] (cm) of children according to recorded daily energy intake (kJ)*

| | Aged 10/11 | | | | | | Aged 14/15 | | | | | |
| | Boys | | | Girls | | | Boys | | | Girls | | |
ENERGY kJ/day	n	mean	sd	n	mean	sd	n	mean	sd	n	mean	sd
4,000 – 5,000	3	138.3	(na)	24	141.9	(na)	3	159.2	(na)	23	159.3	(na)
5,001 – 6,000	20	140.0	7.1	59	140.0	7.1	4	159.5	(na)	44	161.2	6.3
6,001 – 7,000	84	140.1	6.5	176	140.4	6.8	19	163.4	6.1	68	159.3	7.0
7,001 – 8,000	202	141.5	5.7	261	143.0	7.7	50	162.4	8.4	111	160.2	5.3
8,001 – 9,000	239	142.4	6.3	164	143.7	6.7	67	166.5	8.2	96	160.8	6.2
9,001 –10,000	187	143.5	5.1	79	145.8	7.3	90	164.7	7.9	69	163.9	5.7
10,001–11,000	101	145.5	6.5	26	149.6	4.3	78	166.4	8.2	34	162.4	6.4
11,001–12,000	41	147.7	6.3	12	144.1	12.2	84	168.1	7.4	7	161.6	4.4
12,001–13,000	12	146.1	9.6	3	150.2	(na)	57	169.9	8.4	2	158.3	(na)
13,001–14,000	6	139.9	3.0	4	141.5	(na)	30	171.0	7.6	1	166.1	(na)
14,001–15,000	3	152.5	(na)	4	139.5	(na)	17	174.3	5.5	0	–	–
over 15,000	0	–	–	2	146.5	(na)	12	170.1	(na)	0	–	–
	898	142.8	6.1	814	142.9	7.3	511	166.8	8.2	455	161.0	6.1
Standard Height (50th Centile)		139.3			139.5			164.0			161.1	

[1] Height was unavailable for 19 children, (na)=not applicable.

43

Table 7: *Average weights[1] (kg) of children according to recorded daily intake (kJ)*

| | Aged 10/11 | | | | | | Aged 14/15 | | | | | |
| | Boys | | | Girls | | | Boys | | | Girls | | |
ENERGY kJ/day	n	mean	sd	n	mean	sd	n	mean	sd	n	mean	sd
4,000 – 5,000	3	30.3	(na)	23	36.4	(na)	3	63.7	(na)	23	58.7	(na)
5,001 – 6,000	17	38.6	12.4	59	35.9	8.0	4	53.2	(na)	44	56.0	10.0
6,001 – 7,000	82	35.4	8.8	173	35.3	7.8	19	56.5	10.8	68	53.9	8.9
7,001 – 8,000	200	35.5	7.4	258	36.6	7.2	50	57.9	7.1	110	53.5	11.3
8,001 – 9,000	238	36.1	8.2	164	38.2	6.8	65	54.5	10.0	94	51.9	6.5
9,001 –10,000	188	37.1	6.6	79	37.5	6.3	90	54.2	10.2	69	53.3	7.0
10,001–11,000	101	39.0	7.2	26	42.7	5.8	78	55.4	10.4	36	53.3	9.2
11,001–12,000	41	39.8	5.7	12	41.2	11.3	84	56.1	8.3	7	53.7	6.3
12,001–13,000	12	39.0	4.8	3	43.7	(na)	57	57.6	8.8	2	51.8	(na)
13,001–14,000	6	43.8	8.0	4	42.6	(na)	30	58.8	8.1	1	55.0	(na)
14,001–15,000	3	41.0	(na)	4	38.4	(na)	17	62.6	9.6	0	–	–
over 15,000	0	–	–	2	41.2	(na)	12	58.7	(na)	0	–	–
	891	36.8	7.7	807	37.1	7.4	509	55.7	9.5	454	53.7	9.2
Standard Weight (50th Centile)		31.9			33.0			51.9			52.9	

[1] Weight was unavailable for 36 children, (na)=not applicable.

Table 8: *Percentage contribution of specific foods to national average nutrient intakes in Great Britain*

	Boys aged 10/11 years	Girls aged 10/11 years	Boys aged 14/15 years	Girls aged 14/15 years
Number of children	902	821	513	461
Mean energy intakes kJ/day (s.d)	8,670(1,510)	7,690(1,610)	10,400(2,300)	7,850(1,740)
Per cent of energy from:				
Bread	10	9	11	11
Chips	8	8	11	11
Milk	8	7	7	6
Biscuits	7	7	5	5
Other meat products	5	5	6	5
Cake	4	5	4	5
Puddings	5	5	4	4
Other foods	53	54	52	47
Mean fat intakes g/day (s.d)	87.6(17.7)	78.9(18.4)	106.3(27.3)	82.2(20.1)
Per cent of fat from:				
Milk	12	12	10	9
Chips	8	8	11	11
Other meat products	7	7	9	8
Biscuits	8	8	6	6
Carcase meats	6	6	7	7
Crisps	6	7	4	6
Butter	6	6	7	5
Other foods	47	46	46	48
Mean fat intakes as per cent of energy % (s.d)	37.4(3.3)	37.9(3.5)	37.7(3.7)	38.7(3.7)
Contribution to per cent energy from fat from:				
Milk	4	4	4	3
Chips	3	3	4	4
Other meat products	3	3	3	3
Carcase meats	2	2	3	3
Butter	2	2	3	2
Other foods	23	24	21	24
Mean calcium intakes mg/day (s.d)	833(253)	702(217)	925(303)	692(223)
Per cent of calcium from:				
Milk	37	32	33	30
Bread	11	11	14	14
Cheese	8	9	10	10
Puddings	7	7	5	5
Other foods	37	41	38	41

Table 8 (Cont)

	Boys aged 10/11 years	Girls aged 10/11 years	Boys aged 14/15 years	Girls aged 14/15 years
Mean iron intakes mg/day (s.d)	10.0(2.3)	8.6(1.9)	12.2(3.3)	9.3(2.5)
Per cent of iron from:				
Bread	13	13	15	13
Breakfast cereals	13	10	10	8
Chips	6	6	8	8
Other meat products	6	6	7	6
Carcase meats	6	6	6	6
Biscuits	6	6	5	4
Other foods	50	53	49	55
Mean thiamin intakes mg/day (s.d)	1.21(0.35)	1.03(0.31)	1.47(0.49)	1.04(0.31)
Per cent of thiamin from:				
Breakfast cereals	27	23	24	16
Bread	15	14	17	16
Carcase meats	7	8	8	10
Milk	9	8	7	8
Chips	6	6	8	8
Potatoes	5	5	5	6
Other foods	31	36	31	36
Mean riboflavin intakes mg/day (s.d)	1.70(0.59)	1.40(0.47)	1.89(0.72)	1.32(0.50)
Per cent of riboflavin from:				
Milk	30	27	27	30
Breakfast cereals	21	18	19	13
Carcase meats	4	5	5	5
Other foods	45	50	49	52
Mean nicotinic acid equivalent intakes mg/day (s.d)	26.5(5.5)	23.1(5.3)	32.6(8.1)	24.0(5.5)
Per cent of nicotinic acid equivalent from:				
Breakfast cereals	12	8	9	6
Milk	8	7	7	6
Bread	6	6	7	7
Carcase meats	5	5	5	6
Other foods	69	74	72	75
Mean vitamin C intakes mg/day (s.d)	49.3(32.9)	49.0(37.5)	49.3(29.4)	48.0(27.7)
Per cent of vitamin C from:				
Chips	16	16	25	20
Vegetables	15	15	16	19
Potatoes	17	15	17	15
Fruit	13	16	11	14
Fruit Juice	15	15	8	13
Other foods	24	23	23	19

Table 8 (Cont)

	Boys aged 10/11 years	Girls aged 10/11 years	Boys aged 14/15 years	Girls aged 14/15 years
Mean retinol equivalent intakes μg/day (s.d)	845(466)	691(638)	969(1,050)	801(870)
Per cent of retinol equivalent from:				
Carrots	17	19	16	16
Milk	12	11	11	10
Butter	6	7	8	5
Vegetables	6	7	6	8
Cheese	5	6	7	6
Margarine	6	7	5	6
Other foods	48	43	47	49
Mean vitamin D intakes μg/day (s.d)	1.48(1.09)	1.32(0.98)	1.63(1.30)	1.24(0.89)
Per cent of vitamin D from:				
Margarine	24	25	22	27
Eggs	23	21	24	23
Breakfast cereals	16	14	14	9
Other foods	37	40	40	41
Mean pyridoxine intakes mg/day (s.d)	1.17(0.31)	1.03(0.27)	1.35(0.37)	1.06(0.29)
Per cent of pyridoxine from:				
Potatoes	11	11	11	12
Crisps	10	12	7	10
Chips	10	10	14	13
Milk	9	8	8	7
Carcase meats	6	7	7	8
Bread	5	5	6	5
Other foods	49	47	47	45

Table 9: *Percentage contribution of specific foods to average nutrient intakes in Scotland*

	Boys aged 10/11 years	Girls aged 10/11 years	Boys aged 14/15 years	Girls aged 14/15 years
Number of children	457	427	56	42
Mean energy intakes kJ/day (s.d)	8,590(1,380)	7,640(1,370)	10,400(2,030)	8,270(1,740)
Per cent of energy from:				
Bread	10	10	10	11
Chips	8	8	12	11
Milk	10	8	8	6
Biscuits	5	6	5	7
Other meat products	4	4	6	5
Crisps	4	6	3	5
Other foods	59	58	56	55
Mean fat intakes g/day (s.d)	87.2(16.3)	79.0(15.3)	106.6(24.0)	85.7(20.2)
Per cent of fat from:				
Chips	8	8	12	11
Milk	10	8	8	6
Other meat products	7	7	9	7
Crisps	7	9	8	5
Biscuits	6	7	5	8
Carcase meats	6	6	6	6
Butter	6	5	4	6
Other foods	50	57	48	51
Mean fat intakes as per cent of energy % (s.d)	37.6(3.2)	38.3(3.6)	38.0(3.9)	38.3(3.7)
Contribution to per cent of energy from:				
Milk	5	4	4	3
Chips	3	3	5	4
Crisps	3	3	2	4
Other meat products	3	3	3	3
Other foods	24	25	24	24
Mean calcium intakes mg/day (s.d)	876(223)	743(214)	961(325)	725(228)
Per cent of calcium from:				
Milk	40	36	35	30
Bread	10	12	12	13
Cheese	7	8	11	10
Puddings	5	5	4	7
Other foods	38	39	38	40

Table 9 (Cont)

	Boys aged 10/11 years	Girls aged 10/11 years	Boys aged 14/15 years	Girls aged 14/15 years
Mean iron intakes mg/day (s.d)	9.8(2.2)	8.6(2.1)	11.9(3.1)	8.8(1.9)
Per cent of iron from:				
Bread	14	15	15	16
Breakfast cereals	11	7	7	4
Chips	6	6	10	9
Carcase meats	7	7	7	6
Other meat products	5	7	7	6
Other foods	57	58	54	59
Mean thiamin intakes mg/day (s.d)	1.19(0.35)	0.95(0.30)	1.44(0.52)	0.92(0.25)
Per cent of thiamin from:				
Breakfast cereals	27	19	25	12
Bread	15	17	16	19
Milk	10	10	9	8
Carcase meats	7	8	6	11
Chips	6	6	9	4
Other foods	35	40	45	46
Mean riboflavin intakes mg/day (s.d)	1.71(0.54)	1.36(0.45)	1.93(0.72)	1.22(0.40)
Per cent of riboflavin from:				
Milk	34	33	31	30
Breakfast cereals	20	14	25	9
Carcase meats	3	4	3	5
Other foods	43	49	41	56
Mean nicotinic acid equivalent intakes mg/day (s.d)	26.7(5.8)	22.6(4.9)	32.5(7.6)	22.5(5.2)
Per cent of nicotinic acid equivalent from:				
Milk	13	8	7	6
Breakfast cereals	10	8	8	4
Bread	6	6	6	6
Carcase meats	5	5	4	5
Chips	3	3	5	5
Other foods	63	70	70	74
Mean vitamin C intakes mg/day (s.d)	42.5(29.9)	40.6(24.4)	44.7(28.1)	43.1(35.4)
Per cent of vitamin C from:				
Chips	19	17	22	22
Potatoes	17	15	16	14
Fruit	14	18	10	15
Milk	14	11	12	9
Fruit juice	11	13	12	8
Vegetables	10	10	13	9
Other foods	15	16	15	23

49

Table 9 (Cont)

	Boys aged 10/11 years	Girls aged 10/11 years	Boys aged 14/15 years	Girls aged 14/15 years
Mean retinol equivalent intakes µg/day (s.d)	618(703)	586(700)	904(1,303)	513(551)
Per cent of retinol equivalent from:				
Milk	19	16	13	15
Cheese	9	16	9	13
Carrots	10	9	6	7
Butter	8	5	7	11
Margarine	6	7	7	9
Soup	6	7	6	5
Other foods	42	40	52	40
Mean vitamin D intakes µg/day (s.d)	1.24(0.79)	1.15(0.83)	1.76(1.21)	1.09(0.69)
Per cent of vitamin D from:				
Margarine	23	23	26	31
Eggs	25	23	26	25
Breakfast cereals	18	14	15	7
Butter	4	3	2	5
Other foods	30	27	31	32
Mean pyridoxine intakes mg/day (s.d)	1.14(0.32)	0.99(0.24)	1.33(0.35)	1.01(0.25)
Per cent of pyridoxine from:				
Crisps	11	15	9	15
Chips	10	10	16	15
Potatoes	10	10	10	10
Milk	11	10	9	8
Carcase meats	7	7	6	7
Other foods	51	52	50	45

Table 10: *Average daily nutrient intakes of children aged 10/11 years according to region*

Average daily intake of:	Boys				Girls			
	Total Scotland sample	London and SE	North	Rest of GB	Total Scotland sample	London and SE	North	Rest of GB
Energy kJ	8,590	8,790	8,720	8,550	7,640	7,690	7,630	7,770
Protein g	62.2	61.1	61.9	59.9	54.0	52.8	53.7	52.8
Fat g	87.2	88.4	87.6	87.3	79.0	80.1	78.0	78.7
Carbohydrate g	269	280	277	268	237	239	239	247
Calcium mg	880	850	830	810	740	700	710	690
Iron mg	9.8	10.1	10.1	10.0	8.6	8.5	8.6	8.5
Retinol µg	450	580	570	670	430	440	480	460
Carotene µg	1,000	1,560	1,430	1,740	920	1,530	1,390	1,400
Retinol equivalent µg	620	840	810	960	590	700	710	690
Thiamin mg	1.19	1.21	1.24	1.18	0.95	1.02	1.06	1.04
Riboflavin mg	1.71	1.69	1.75	1.66	1.36	1.38	1.45	1.37
Nicotinic acid mg	14.5	14.6	15.4	14.2	11.9	12.4	13.1	12.6
Nicotinic acid equiv-alent mg	26.7	26.4	27.4	25.9	22.6	22.7	23.6	22.9
Vitamin C mg	42.5	55.5	43.6	51.2	40.6	56.2	44.1	50.5
Vitamin D µg	1.24	1.40	1.54	1.54	1.15	1.24	1.36	1.40
Pyridoxine mg	1.14	1.19	1.17	1.67	0.99	1.04	1.07	1.00
Height cm (s.d)	142.5(6.3)	142.9(5.9)	142.9(6.4)	142.5(6.6)	142.9(7.3)	142.4(7.4)	142.9(7.8)	143.2(7.1)
Base	457	238	260	317	424	217	262	257

Table 11: *Average daily nutrient intakes of children aged 14/15 years according to region*

Average daily intake of:	Boys				Girls			
	Scotland	London and SE	North	Rest of GB	Scotland	London and SE	North	Rest of GB
Energy kJ	10,400	10,210	10,510	10,460	8,270	7,680	7,960	7,790
Protein g	74.8	74.4	74.7	74.7	55.9	55.9	57.3	55.7
Fat g	106.6	105.1	107.7	105.8	85.7	80.1	83.4	81.6
Carbohydrate g	323	314	328	328	259	234	242	238
Calcium mg	960	920	900	940	720	660	609	710
Iron mg	11.9	12.2	12.3	12.2	8.8	9.4	9.5	9.1
Retinol µg	720	750	690	640	360	560	680	510
Carotene µg	1,120	1,750	1,760	1,620	920	1,470	1,620	1,450
Retinol equivalent µg	900	1,040	990	910	510	800	950	750
Thiamin mg	1.44	1.47	1.44	1.50	0.92	1.03	1.06	1.06
Riboflavin mg	1.93	1.87	1.86	1.92	1.22	1.31	1.36	1.33
Nicotinic acid mg	18.2	18.1	18.1	18.6	11.6	13.1	13.4	12.8
Nicotinic acid equivalent mg	32.5	32.5	32.5	32.9	22.5	24.0	24.8	23.7
Vitamin C mg	44.7	52.1	46.1	51.4	43.1	52.4	44.8	49.2
Vitamin D µg	1.76	1.48	1.69	1.66	1.09	1.14	1.33	1.27
Pyridoxine mg	1.33	1.33	1.33	1.38	1.01	1.07	1.07	1.02
Height cm (s.d)	167.4(8.6)	167.0(9.2)	166.2(7.9)	167.0(7.8)	161.2(6.1)	161.6(6.4)	160.4(6.0)	160.9(6.1)
Base	56	145	149	162	42	129	122	164

52

Table 12: *Daily intake of energy and nutrients by social class and employment status among 10/11 year old boys from two parent families*

Average daily intake of:	Father working — social class:						Father unemployed or long-term sick	Father employed
	I	II	III non-manual	III manual	IV	V		
Energy kJ	8,560	8,960	8,060	8,710	8,460	8,380	8,820	8,660
Protein g	68.3	62.4	60.8	60.4	58.1	57.6	60.6	61.3
Fat g	87.3	91.5	81.0	88.0	84.4	82.8	90.1	87.6
Carbohydrate g	260	281	252	276	271	270	278	273
Calcium mg	930	910	770	810	820	810	790	850
Iron mg	10.0	11.3	10.4	9.6	9.3	9.3	10.0	10.0
Retinol μg	750	560	920	560	540	590	420	620
Carotene μg	1,670	1,710	1,260	1,510	1,390	1,700	1,590	1,550
Retinol equivalent μg	1,030	840	1,130	810	770	870	690	870
Thiamin mg	1.34	1.24	1.16	1.22	1.29	1.16	1.19	1.22
Riboflavin mg	1.95	1.83	1.72	1.64	1.64	1.61	1.56	1.74
Nicotinic acid mg	16.3	15.0	15.0	14.6	14.3	13.9	14.2	14.8
Nicotinic acid equivalent mg	29.4	27.0	26.8	26.3	25.7	25.1	26.1	26.7
Vitamin C mg	58.7	61.1	45.6	46.4	37.8	46.3	39.5	51.0
Vitamin D μg	1.73	1.53	1.49	1.40	1.48	1.15	1.54	1.47
Pyridoxine mg	1.20	1.20	1.32	1.16	1.12	1.07	1.10	1.18
Height cm (s.d)	147.4(6.1)	143.7(5.6)	144.7(6.3)	141.9(6.3)	142.6(7.7)	140.2(5.9)	140.8(5.5)	143.2(6.2)
Base (weighted)	48	220	84	219	76	30	123	677

53

Table 13: *Daily intake of energy and nutrients by social class and employment status among 10/11 year old girls from two parent families*

Average daily intake of:	Father working — social class: I	II	III non-manual	III manual	IV	V	Father unemployed or long-term sick	Father employed
Energy kJ	7,220	7,720	7,630	7,790	7,720	7,670	7,640	7,680
Protein g	53.4	54.4	53.2	52.9	52.8	53.8	51.3	53.4
Fat g	73.6	78.7	78.1	79.5	79.9	79.5	77.8	78.6
Carbohydrate g	224	242	239	247	241	239	243	241
Calcium mg	740	740	740	700	660	680	650	710
Iron mg	8.4	8.7	8.5	8.7	8.4	9.0	8.4	8.6
Retinol μg	640	440	560	440	470	670	380	490
Carotene μg	1,690	1,520	1,600	1,230	1,310	1,020	1,280	1,420
Retinol equivalent μg	920	690	830	640	690	850	600	730
Thiamin mg	1.05	1.05	1.09	1.05	1.01	0.97	1.00	1.05
Riboflavin mg	1.54	1.49	1.51	1.39	1.31	1.33	1.27	1.44
Nicotinic acid mg	12.9	13.1	12.9	12.9	12.2	12.1	12.3	12.8
Nicotinic acid equivalent mg	23.4	23.6	23.2	23.2	22.6	22.9	22.4	23.3
Vitamin C mg	51.8	63.2	60.7	45.5	39.3	44.4	36.7	53.3
Vitamin D μg	1.30	1.35	1.15	1.25	1.33	1.65	1.40	1.29
Pyridoxine mg	1.09	1.05	1.05	1.02	1.02	1.01	0.98	1.04
Height cm (s.d)	142.0(8.1)	143.4(8.2)	144.0(7.2)	143.6(6.7)	143.7(7.5)	140.2(6.2)	140.8(6.6)	143.3(7.5)
Base (weighted)	51	182	93	157	70	25	128	578

Table 14: *Daily intake of energy and nutrients by social class and employment status among 14/15 year old boys from two parent families*

Average daily intake of:	Father working – social class:						Father unemployed or long-term sick	Father employed
	I	II	III non-manual	III manual	IV	V		
Energy kJ	11,300	11,250	11,440	10,420	10,260	(9,460)	10,100	10,490
Protein g	80.8	76.0	84.1	74.6	71.9	(71.3)	71.4	75.9
Fat g	116.7	105.8	120.6	106.2	102.9	(98.2)	102.3	107.5
Carbohydrate g	347	314	346	325	326	(288)	318	325
Calcium mg	1,100	970	1,050	930	870	(760)	830	950
Iron mg	14.1	11.9	13.1	12.2	12.1	(12.2)	11.8	12.3
Retinol µg	890	840	1,020	640	630	(480)	500	740
Carotene µg	2,240	1,830	1,650	1,670	1,360	(1,810)	1,540	1,720
Retinol equivalent µg	1,030	1,270	1,290	920	850	(780)	750	1,030
Thiamin mg	1.83	1.40	1.55	1.51	1.44	(1.29)	1.34	1.49
Riboflavin mg	2.41	1.94	2.10	1.93	1.75	(1.61)	1.69	1.96
Nicotinic acid mg	22.3	17.9	19.3	18.7	17.6	(17.6)	16.9	18.6
Nicotinic acid equivalent mg	37.7	32.5	35.5	33.0	31.6	(31.6)	30.6	33.2
Vitamin C mg	65.9	58.0	49.3	48.3	40.5	(49.4)	40.5	51.5
Vitamin D µg	1.62	1.97	2.00	1.57	1.14	(1.54)	1.58	1.62
Pyridoxine mg	1.40	1.33	1.35	1.38	1.30	(1.42)	1.32	1.36
Height cm (s.d)	168.8(9.5)	167.4(7.6)	168.3(9.7)	167.5(8.3)	165.5(9.0)	164.6(9.0)	165.0(7.8)	167.2(8.4)
Base	33	103	32	125	59	(11)	69	363

55

Table 15: *Daily intake of energy and nutrients by social class and employment status among 14/15 year old girls from two parent families*

Average daily intake of:	Father working – social class:						Father unemployed or long-term sick	Father employed
	I	II	III non-manual	III manual	IV	V		
Energy kJ	7,679	7,930	7,600	8,020	7,710	(7,490)	7,950	7,830
Protein g	58.9	57.9	52.0	58.5	54.6	(54.7)	55.6	56.5
Fat g	84.0	85.5	78.9	83.4	80.7	(78.5)	82.5	82.4
Carbohydrate g	222	236	237	245	236	(228)	245	238
Calcium mg	730	750	670	720	660	(600)	680	700
Iron mg	10.4	9.5	9.1	9.3	8.8	(9.2)	9.3	9.3
Retinol µg	990	590	470	570	380	(640)	640	560
Carotene µg	2,750	1,410	1,260	1,480	1,250	(1,180)	1,400	1,470
Retinol equivalent µg	1,450	830	680	810	590	(840)	870	800
Thiamin mg	1.11	1.05	1.04	1.08	1.01	(1.01)	1.01	1.05
Riboflavin mg	1.55	1.38	1.30	1.38	1.24	(1.18)	1.26	1.34
Nicotinic acid mg	14.7	13.2	12.3	13.4	12.7	(12.3)	12.5	13.1
Nicotinic acid equivalent mg	26.2	24.4	22.5	24.9	23.3	(23.0)	23.4	24.1
Vitamin C mg	60.2	49.6	43.0	46.9	50.3	(37.3)	43.8	49.1
Vitamin D µg	1.32	1.39	1.19	1.31	1.10	(1.19)	1.25	1.26
Pyridoxine mg	1.10	1.06	1.02	1.08	1.07	(1.01)	1.03	1.07
Height cm (s.d)	163.0(6.0)	161.3(6.3)	161.7(6.9)	161.7(6.0)	160.5(5.9)	160.1(5.1)	159.7(6.5)	161.4(6.1)
Base	25	70	44	94	64	(15)	70	312

56

Table 16: *Daily intake of energy and nutrients by family composition among 10/11 year old boys*

Average daily intake of:	One parent families			Two parent families			
	One child	Two or more children	All one parent families	One child	Two children	Three children	Four or more children
Energy kJ	8,750	8,430	8,520	8,610	8,760	8,500	8,800
Protein g	61.1	58.9	59.2	60.1	62.0	60.3	59.8
Fat g	84.4	83.7	83.9	87.9	88.4	87.1	89.2
Carbohydrate g	286	271	275	271	277	265	280
Calcium mg	790	790	790	780	860	850	770
Iron mg	10.4	10.2	10.2	9.6	10.2	9.8	9.9
Retinol µg	630	680	660	520	600	580	620
Carotene µg	1,280	1,210	1,220	1,410	1,550	1,470	1,210
Retinol requivalent µg	840	880	860	750	860	830	980
Thiamin mg	1.22	1.19	1.19	1.14	1.23	1.19	1.29
Riboflavin mg	1.67	1.65	1.64	1.52	1.75	1.71	1.65
Nicotinic acid mg	15.2	14.3	14.4	14.0	15.0	14.2	15.3
Nicotinic acid equivalent mg	27.1	25.7	25.9	25.8	27.0	25.9	26.9
Vitamin C mg	60.0	44.5	49.4	52.5	51.0	47.6	38.5
Vitamin D µg	1.25	1.58	1.44	1.42	1.51	1.44	1.53
Pyridoxine mg	1.16	1.13	1.13	1.19	1.19	1.14	1.15
Height cm (s.d)	143.7(6.1)	141.7(7.4)	141.9(6.5)	143.7(6.5)	143.5(6.2)	141.9(6.1)	140.7(5.2)
Base (weighted)	34	71	105	91	447	188	73

57

Table 17: *Daily intake of energy and nutrients by family composition among 10/11 year old girls*

Average daily intake of:	One parent families			Two parent families			
	One child	Two or more children	All one parent families	One child	Two children	Three children	Four or more children
Energy kJ	7,660	8,100	8,020	7,520	7,690	7,820	7,270
Protein g	54.3	55.6	55.3	53.9	52.6	52.6	53.1
Fat g	80.2	84.1	83.3	77.7	78.9	79.7	72.5
Carbohydrate g	235	253	250	233	242	248	230
Calcium mg	640	730	710	730	690	690	720
Iron mg	8.6	8.9	8.8	8.8	8.5	8.4	8.5
Retinol µg	490	350	380	460	500	470	340
Carotene µg	1,500	1,400	1,420	1,570	1,270	1,410	1,570
Retinol equivalent µg	740	590	610	730	720	710	600
Thiamin mg	0.85	1.07	1.02	1.00	1.03	1.05	1.14
Riboflavin mg	1.16	1.40	1.35	1.41	1.39	1.38	1.52
Nicotinic acid mg	11.7	12.7	12.5	12.6	12.6	12.8	13.2
Nicotinic acid equivalent mg	22.5	23.6	23.4	22.9	22.9	23.1	23.4
Vitamin C mg	39.7	40.5	40.3	56.5	53.4	46.6	31.9
Vitamin D µg	1.31	1.50	1.46	1.24	1.26	1.52	1.21
Pyridoxine mg	1.02	1.07	1.06	1.11	1.03	1.01	0.92
Height cm (s.d)	147.9(6.6)	142.2(6.6)	143.5(7.1)	145.5(8.8)	142.6(6.8)	142.9(7.6)	139.2(5.8)
Base (weighted)	21	88	110	120	337	141	73

Table 18: *Daily intake of energy and nutrients by family composition among 14/15 year old boys*

Average daily intake of:	One parent families			Two parent families			
	One child	Two or more children	All one parent families	One child	Two children	Three children	Four or more children
Energy kJ	10,900	9,460	10,340	10.710	10,680	10,690	10.400
Protein g	76.4	67.2	72.8	74.2	76.0	76.7	72.2
Fat g	111.2	96.6	105.5	104.2	108.4	108.5	108.5
Carbohydrate g	341	296	323	314	335	335	324
Calcium mg	950	780	880	900	990	960	850
Iron mg	12.7	11.3	12.1	12.0	12.4	12.4	12.1
Retinol µg	620	780	680	720	710	580	760
Carotene µg	1,490	1,690	1,570	1,690	1,710	1,650	1,350
Retinol equivalent µg	860	1,060	940	1,000	990	850	980
Thiamin mg	1.52	1.31	1.44	1.47	1.48	1.54	1.34
Riboflavin mg	1.97	1.65	1.85	1.85	2.01	1.97	1.67
Nicotinic acid mg	19.3	16.7	18.3	18.4	18.4	18.8	16.4
Nicotinic acid equivalent mg	33.9	29.8	32.3	32.7	32.9	33.5	30.4
Vitamin C mg	53.6	38.6	47.7	48.2	54.8	49.1	39.8
Vitamin D µg	1.78	1.71	1.75	1.55	1.66	1.56	1.83
Pyridoxine mg	1.38	1.25	1.33	1.34	1.37	1.40	1.21
Height cm (s.d)	166.2(8.0)	166.2(8.3)	166.0(7.8)	167.2(8.0)	166.7(8.9)	167.1(8.8)	166.5(8.6)
Base	49	31	80	207	131	58	37

Table 19: *Daily intake of energy and nutrients by family composition among 14/15 year old girls*

Average daily intake of:	One parent families			Two parent families			
	One child	Two or more children	All one parent families	One child	Two children	Three children	Four or more children
Energy kJ	7,880	7,910	7,940	7,830	7,680	8,140	8,120
Protein g	55.9	56.0	56.1	57.2	55.5	56.1	55.0
Fat g	81.6	82.3	82.2	82.5	81.2	83.8	83.0
Carbohydrate g	243	243	245	237	232	255	257
Calcium mg	650	690	670	710	690	690	640
Iron mg	9.1	9.3	9.2	9.3	9.1	9.7	9.3
Retinol μg	390	460	410	560	570	670	590
Carotene μg	1,320	1,390	1,330	1,600	1,460	1,190	1,300
Retinol equivalent μg	610	690	630	830	820	870	810
Thiamin mg	1.02	0.99	1.01	1.01	1.07	1.09	1.05
Riboflavin mg	1.26	1.24	1.25	1.32	1.38	1.30	1.27
Nicotinic acid mg	12.8	12.6	12.3	12.6	13.3	13.1	13.7
Nicotinic acid equivalent mg	23.8	23.6	23.8	23.8	24.1	24.1	24.6
Vitamin C mg	50.0	47.3	48.7	48.5	48.9	46.6	42.8
Vitamin D μg	1.14	1.16	1.14	1.15	1.28	1.36	1.41
Pyridoxine mg	1.11	1.07	1.09	1.07	1.05	1.06	1.10
Height cm (s.d)	161.3(6.4)	160.7(6.4)	161.0(6.2)	160.7(5.9)	161.3(6.0)	162.6(4.8)	158.2(8.6)
Base	38	33	75	159	142	52	35

Table 20: *Daily intake of energy and nutrients by receipt of benefits among 10/11 year olds*

Boys Average daily intake of:	Family receiving		Neither of these
	Family Income Supplement	Supplementary Benefit (or both)	
Energy kJ	8,350	8,770	8,640
Protein g	56.5	58.7	61.4
Fat g	81.9	88.6	87.5
Carbohydrate g	272	281	272
Calcium mg	700	780	840
Iron mg	10.2	10.0	10.0
Retinol μg	820	530	600
Carotene μg	1,190	1,500	1,550
Retinol equivalent μg	1,020	780	850
Thiamin mg	1.23	1.18	1.21
Riboflavin mg	1.68	1.53	1.72
Nicotinic acid mg	15.5	14.0	14.7
Nicotinic acid equivalent mg	26.5	25.5	26.6
Vitamin C mg	54.0	40.1	51.0
Vitamin D μg	1.56	1.54	1.46
Pyridoxine mg	1.17	1.14	1.18
Height cm (s.d)	140.8(5.4)	140.4(5.8)	143.3(6.2)
Base (weighted)	32	135	728
Girls Average daily intake of:			
Energy kJ	7,350	7,650	7,720
Protein g	54.6	52.6	53.3
Fat g	75.3	79.2	79.0
Carbohydrate g	227	239	243
Calcium mg	640	660	710
Iron mg	8.0	8.4	8.6
Retinol μg	320	580	480
Carotene μg	1,210	1,360	1,390
Retinol equivalent μg	530	610	720
Thiamin mg	1.00	1.02	1.04
Riboflavin mg	1.22	1.32	1.42
Nicotinic acid mg	12.3	12.5	12.7
Nicotinic acid equivalent mg	23.1	22.9	23.1
Vitamin C mg	43.0	37.1	51.9
Vitamin D μg	1.54	1.31	1.32
Pyridoxine mg	1.04	1.01	1.04
Height cm (s.d)	144.2(8.3)	140.6(6.9)	143.3(7.3)
Base (weighted)	26	138	641

Table 21: *Daily intake of energy and nutrients by receipt of benefits among 14/15 year olds*

Boys Average daily intake of:	Family receiving		Neither of these
	Family Income Supplement	Supplementary Benefit (or both)	
Energy kJ	(9,810)	9,890	10,480
Protein g	(67.9)	68.8	75.8
Fat g	(101.7)	101.6	107.0
Carbohydrate g	(304)	311	325
Calcium mg	(820)	820	940
Iron mg	(10.5)	11.5	12.4
Retinol μg	(320)	690	710
Carotene μg	(1,560)	1,610	1,650
Retinol equivalent μg	(580)	960	980
Thiamin mg	(1.45)	1.34	1.49
Riboflavin mg	(1.56)	1.69	1.94
Nicotinic acid mg	(17.6)	16.6	13.2
Nicotinic acid equivalent mg	(30.7)	29.8	33.2
Vitamin C mg	(40.3)	40.1	51.7
Vitamin D μg	(1.85)	1.40	1.65
Pyridoxine mg	(1.19)	1.26	1.37
Height cm (s.d)	166.9(8.5)	164.3(8.2)	167.2(8.2)
Base	(15)	68	444

Girls Average daily intake of:			
Energy kJ	(8,270)	8,250	7,760
Protein g	(56.4)	56.5	56.1
Fat g	(86.7)	85.5	81.4
Carbohydrate g	(254)	256	236
Calcium mg	(700)	820	940
Iron mg	(9.6)	9.8	9.2
Retinol μg	(260)	720	540
Carotene μg	(1,400)	1,370	1,490
Retinol equivalent μg	(490)	950	790
Thiamin mg	(1.05)	1.03	1.04
Riboflavin mg	(1.21)	1.31	1.33
Nicotinic acid mg	(12.8)	12.9	13.0
Nicotinic acid equivalent mg	(23.9)	24.1	23.9
Vitamin C mg	(47.6)	44.2	48.9
Vitamin D μg	(1.30)	1.23	1.24
Pyridoxine mg	(1.07)	1.09	1.06
Height cm (s.d)	159.5(5.7)	159.9(6.5)	161.2(6.0)
Base	(10)	71	368

Table 22: *Average daily nutrient intakes of boys aged 10/11 years according to lunchtime meal*

Average daily intake of:	Paid school meal	Free school meal	Paid school meal most days	Free school meal most days	Home	Packed lunch	Cafe
Energy kJ	8,850	8,810	8,550	8,500	8,430	8,680	(9,470)
Protein g	62.2	60.4	59.8	58.5	59.2	61.5	(69.7)
Fat g	89.3	89.3	86.3	83.5	83.5	88.8	(99.5)
Carbohydrate g	279	280	271	270	270	271	(287)
Calcium mg	810	800	790	730	790	870	(900)
Iron mg	9.4	9.3	9.7	9.6	9.9	10.0	(11.2)
Retinol μg	720	520	580	850	560	490	(800)
Carotene μg	1,870	1,670	1,280	1,000	1,340	1,500	(1,490)
Retinol equivalent μg	1,030	800	790	1,010	780	740	(1,040)
Thiamin mg	1.26	1.20	1.13	1.25	1.16	1.22	(1.33)
Riboflavin mg	1.85	1.63	1.62	1.66	1.58	1.70	(1.86)
Nicotinic acid mg	15.2	14.4	14.4	15.3	14.0	14.6	(15.9)
Nicotinic acid equivalent mg	27.2	26.2	25.9	26.5	25.5	26.7	(29.3)
Vitamin C mg	52.2	40.8	49.3	38.0	45.7	55.5	(49.0)
Vitamin D μg	1.28	1.56	1.47	1.39	1.46	1.68	(1.46)
Pyridoxine mg	1.25	1.17	1.13	1.15	1.11	1.15	(1.31)
Height cm (s.d)	143.7(6.7)	140.7(5.8)	144.4(4.9)	141.0(5.8)	142.0(6.5)	142.9(6.5)	142.9(4.7)
Base (weighted)	227	127	97	46	133	256	(20)

Table 23: *Average daily nutrient intakes of girls aged 10/11 years according to lunchtime meal*

Average daily intake of:	Paid school meal	Free school meal	Paid school meal most days	Free school meal most days	Home	Packed lunch	Cafe
Energy kJ	7,630	7,540	7,750	7,350	7,350	7,790	(9,470)
Protein g	54.6	50.8	53.3	52.3	55.5	52.8	(69.7)
Fat g	79.8	77.9	78.5	76.6	79.3	79.1	(99.5)
Carbohydrate g	234	237	246	226	249	247	(287)
Calcium mg	720	650	670	680	750	720	(900)
Iron mg	8.5	8.3	8.7	8.2	8.9	8.6	(11.2)
Retinol µg	460	430	360	460	490	470	(800)
Carotene µg	1,390	1,510	1,380	1,160	1,280	1,410	(1,490)
Retinol equivalent µg	690	680	590	650	700	700	(1,040)
Thiamin mg	1.02	0.98	1.07	1.25	0.92	1.07	(1.33)
Riboflavin mg	1.45	1.27	1.36	1.26	1.46	1.44	(1.86)
Nicotinic acid mg	12.7	11.9	13.3	11.9	12.6	12.0	(15.9)
Nicotinic acid equivalent mg	23.2	21.9	23.8	22.2	23.5	23.3	(29.3)
Vitamin C mg	51.6	36.8	51.0	36.4	44.7	51.1	(49.0)
Vitamin D µg	1.07	1.32	1.21	1.28	1.62	1.44	(1.46)
Pyridoxine mg	1.02	0.99	1.09	0.98	1.06	1.04	(1.31)
Height cm (s.d)	142.8(8.8)	140.4(6.5)	143.6(5.8)	142.5(7.6)	144.2(7.0)	142.9(7.0)	142.9(4.7)
Base (weighted)	196	137	75	32	109	263	(20)

Table 24: *Average daily nutrient intakes of boys aged 14/15 years according to lunchtime meal*

Average daily intake of:	Paid school meal	Free school meal	Paid school meal most days	Free school meal most days	Home	Packed lunch	Cafe
Energy kJ	10,450	10,590	10,410	10,120	10,220	10,700	10,370
Protein g	74.6	72.1	72.3	72.3	74.6	79.4	72.6
Fat g	105.3	111.0	105.8	99.6	104.1	110.3	106.3
Carbohydrate g	329	329	327	311	318	327	324
Calcium mg	950	860	920	800	930	1,020	870
Iron mg	12.2	12.2	12.0	11.6	11.8	12.0	11.9
Retinol µg	650	540	380	930	690	1,110	390
Carotene µg	1,710	1,540	1,460	1,340	1,650	1,990	1,430
Retinol equivalent µg	940	790	620	1,160	960	1,440	630
Thiamin mg	1.44	1.35	1.44	1.42	1.49	1.02	1.35
Riboflavin mg	1.86	1.60	1.82	1.85	1.94	2.15	1.76
Nicotinic acid mg	17.5	16.4	17.5	18.3	18.6	20.3	17.5
Nicotinic acid equivalent mg	31.9	30.6	31.4	32.0	32.7	35.6	31.5
Vitamin C mg	57.9	41.0	56.9	40.1	40.6	56.6	44.5
Vitamin D µg	1.35	1.61	1.35	1.97	1.53	2.13	1.60
Pyridoxine mg	1.24	1.26	1.37	1.38	1.32	1.39	1.32
Height cm (s.d)	166.2(7.8)	165.6(9.1)	167.1(8.3)	165.2(8.5)	168.0(8.3)	166.6(8.4)	167.4(7.6)
Base	86	50	58	25	119	105	68

Table 25: *Average daily nutrient intakes of girls aged 14/15 years according to lunchtime meal*

Average daily intake of:	Paid school meal	Free school meal	Paid school meal most days	Free school meal most days	Home	Packed lunch	Cafe
Energy kJ	8,060	8,560	8,040	(8,220)	7,410	7,880	7,710
Protein g	56.1	56.4	56.4	(55.7)	54.8	59.1	51.9
Fat g	85.9	89.5	85.1	(82.0)	77.1	82.7	79.6
Carbohydrate g	244	268	244	(264)	225	238	241
Calcium mg	690	680	720	(680)	670	730	650
Iron mg	9.2	9.7	9.3	(9.4)	8.9	9.9	8.5
Retinol µg	520	490	420	(360)	590	740	440
Carotene µg	1,500	1,390	1,380	(1,260)	1,400	1,670	1,110
Retinol equivalent µg	770	720	650	(570)	830	1,020	620
Thiamin mg	1.04	1.02	1.04	(1.07)	0.97	1.11	1.03
Riboflavin mg	1.30	1.22	1.37	(1.28)	1.28	1.44	1.24
Nicotinic acid mg	12.5	12.5	12.9	(13.5)	12.3	14.0	12.7
Nicotinic acid equivalent mg	23.7	23.7	24.3	(24.5)	23.0	25.6	22.8
Vitamin C mg	50.7	41.0	51.2	(44.2)	41.2	55.9	46.1
Vitamin D µg	1.05	1.17	1.17	(1.19)	1.30	1.50	0.97
Pyridoxine mg	1.07	1.08	1.08	(1.05)	1.02	1.08	1.07
Height cm (s.d)	160.0(6.4)	158.5(8.0)	161.2(6.3)	160.3(5.5)	160.7(5.7)	162.4(5.9)	160.9(4.9)
Base	72	38	56	(19)	101	121	54

Table 26: *Average weekday lunchtime intakes of 10/11 year old boys*

Average lunchtime intake of:	Paid school meal	Free school meal	Paid school meal most days	Free school meal most days	Home	Packed lunch	Cafe
Energy kJ	2,710	2,760	2,520	2,600	2,660	2,700	(2,690)
Per cent daily energy intake (5 day)	30	31	29	30	31	31	(28)
Protein g	19.2	19.0	17.2	18.1	18.6	16.9	(20.3)
Fat g	29.9	30.7	27.8	28.6	27.1	30.6	(29.5)
Fat as per cent of energy	41	45	41	41	38	42	(41)
Carbohydrate g	80	82	75	97	84	80	(78)
Calcium mg	230	250	200	200	230	250	(210)
Iron mg	2.9	2.9	2.9	2.9	3.1	3.0	(3.5)
Retinol μg	160	60	320	230	98	160	(250)
Carotene μg	970	690	390	350	440	140	(130)
Retinol equivalent μg	320	180	390	290	170	180	(290)
Thiamin mg	0.26	0.26	0.24	0.25	0.29	0.27	(0.29)
Riboflavin mg	0.35	0.35	0.33	0.33	0.32	0.28	(0.34)
Nicotinic acid mg	3.2	3.1	3.2	3.1	3.3	3.2	(2.8)
Nicotinic acid equivalent mg	7.0	6.8	6.8	6.8	7.0	6.8	(7.7)
Vitamin C mg	15.9	12.6	12.8	12.9	17.5	16.6	(12.1)
Vitamin D μg	0.21	0.23	0.28	0.29	0.44	0.79	(0.33)
Pyridoxine mg	0.35	0.34	0.33	0.32	0.31	0.29	(0.23)
Base (weighted)	227	127	97	46	133	256	(20)

Table 27: *Average weekday lunchtime intakes of 10/11 year old girls*

Average lunchtime intake of:	Paid school meal	Free school meal	Paid school meal most days	Free school meal most days	Home	Packed lunch	Cafe
Energy kJ	2,280	2,360	2,400	2,320	2,360	2,700	(2,500)
Per cent of daily energy intake (5 day)	30	31	31	32	30	33	(33)
Protein g	16.0	16.2	16.8	16.7	17.3	14.5	(15.4)
Fat g	25.7	26.2	26.1	25.3	24.2	28.0	(28.2)
Fat as per cent of energy	42	41	40	40	38	41	(42)
Carbohydrate g	66	65	74	68	73	78	(75)
Calcium mg	180	210	190	210	210	200	(160)
Iron mg	2.5	2.4	2.9	2.5	3.1	2.7	(2.7)
Retinol μg	120	120	77	130	220	210	(60)
Carotene μg	520	840	500	580	410	230	(240)
Retinol equivalent μg	200	260	160	230	290	240	(100)
Thiamin mg	0.21	0.23	0.24	0.22	0.27	0.26	(0.25)
Riboflavin mg	0.28	0.30	0.28	0.32	0.36	0.23	(0.24)
Nicotinic acid mg	2.7	2.7	2.9	2.9	3.1	3.0	(2.3)
Nicotinic acid equivalent mg	6.0	6.0	6.3	6.2	6.8	6.0	(6.1)
Vitamin C mg	11.3	11.2	13.2	12.0	12.5	18.8	(15.2)
Vitamin D μg	0.19	0.25	0.25	0.19	0.42	0.67	(0.33)
Pyridoxine mg	0.30	0.29	0.32	0.30	0.29	0.28	(0.33)
Base (weighted)	196	137	75	32	109	263	(20)

Table 28: *Average weekday lunchtime intakes of 14/15 year old boys*

Average lunchtime intake of:	Paid school meal	Free school meal	Paid school meal most days	Free school meal most days	Home	Packed lunch	Cafe
Energy kJ	3,720	4,170	3,480	3,510	3,290	3,280	3,450
Per cent of daily energy intake (5 day)	36	39	22	25	32	31	33
Protein g	22.7	24.4	21.1	23.3	24.4	23.5	18.4
Fat g	39.5	45.8	38.3	37.8	35.7	37.8	38.1
Fat as per cent of energy	39	41	41	40	40	43	41
Carbohydrate g	117	129	107	107	97	98	108
Calcium mg	260	300	240	260	290	310	190
Iron mg	4.2	4.4	3.8	3.9	4.0	4.0	3.5
Retinol μg	92	67	78	200	200	250	50
Carotene μg	150	260	110	550	380	110	110
Retinol equivalent μg	170	110	96	290	270	270	69
Thiamin mg	0.35	0.37	0.31	0.32	0.38	0.42	0.31
Riboflavin mg	0.34	0.37	0.31	0.35	0.43	0.35	0.25
Nicotinic acid mg	4.2	4.2	4.2	4.3	4.5	4.8	3.8
Nicotinic acid equivalent mg	8.9	9.3	8.5	9.4	9.4	9.7	7.5
Vitamin C mg	17.0	15.9	14.8	14.5	9.3	12.7	16.3
Vitamin D μg	0.18	0.27	0.26	0.32	0.57	1.00	0.22
Pyridoxine mg	0.44	0.48	0.41	0.44	0.38	0.32	0.39
Base	86	50	58	25	119	105	68

Table 29: *Average weekday lunchtime intakes of 14/15 year old girls*

Average lunchtime intake of:	Paid school meal	Free school meal	Paid school meal most days	Free school meal most days	Home	Packed lunch	Cafe
Energy kJ	3,110	3,660	2,870	(3,090)	2,340	2,420	2,440
Per cent of daily energy intake (5 day)	39	43	36	(38)	32	31	32
Protein g	17.7	20.7	17.0	(19.4)	17.1	16.6	12.2
Fat g	34.9	39.3	31.9	(34.3)	24.7	26.4	26.7
Fat as per cent of energy	41	40	41	(41)	39	40	40
Carbohydrate g	95	116	88	(93)	71	73	78
Calcium mg	200	250	210	(210)	210	220	140
Iron mg	3.3	3.8	3.2	(3.4)	3.0	2.9	2.4
Retinol µg	55	62	160	(61)	200	230	33
Carotene µg	240	190	300	(180)	260	160	150
Retinol equivalent µg	95	93	210	(91)	240	250	58
Thiamin mg	0.30	0.34	0.27	(0.27)	0.31	0.31	0.23
Riboflavin mg	0.25	0.32	0.29	(0.26)	0.31	0.28	0.17
Nicotinic acid mg	3.3	3.8	3.3	(3.4)	3.1	3.5	2.7
Nicotinic acid equivalent mg	7.0	8.1	6.9	(7.2)	6.6	6.9	5.2
Vitamin C mg	16.6	18.2	12.3	(12.3)	9.7	12.6	13.7
Vitamin D µg	0.23	0.25	0.31	(0.28)	0.41	0.74	0.20
Pyridoxine mg	0.37	0.43	0.34	(0.38)	0.28	0.27	0.29
Base	72	38	56	(19)	101	121	54

Table 30: *Average weekday lunchtime intakes of 10/11 year old boys in Scotland*

Average lunchtime intake of:	Paid school meal	Free school meal	Paid school meal most days	Free school meal most days	Home	Packed lunch
Energy kJ	2,570	2,670	2,470	(2,330)	2,420	2,640
Per cent of daily energy intake (5 day)	29	31	31	(26)	29	33
Protein g	19.5	20.2	17.9	(17.3)	17.5	16.6
Fat g	28.5	29.4	28.2	(25.4)	24.8	27.5
Fat as per cent of energy	41	41	42	(40)	38	39
Carbohydrate g	74	77	70	(69)	75	84
Calcium mg	250	300	210	(240)	260	250
Iron mg	2.8	2.7	2.8	(2.4)	2.9	2.9
Retinol μg	80	70	60	(80)	100	100
Carotene μg	440	440	430	(140)	250	220
Retinol equivalent μg	160	140	130	(110)	150	140
Thiamin mg	0.24	0.25	0.22	(0.22)	0.27	0.31
Riboflavin mg	0.37	0.43	0.30	(0.34)	0.35	0.27
Nicotinic acid mg	3.1	2.9	3.1	(2.6)	2.9	3.1
Nicotinic acid equivalent mg	7.0	7.1	6.7	(6.2)	6.5	6.5
Vitamin C mg	11.2	11.8	10.4	(9.4)	9.7	10.1
Vitamin D μg	0.16	0.23	0.20	(0.31)	0.41	0.33
Pyridoxine mg	0.32	0.33	0.30	(0.28)	0.27	0.25
Base	65	75	49	(19)	200	37

Table 31: *Average weekday lunchtime intakes of 10/11 year old girls in Scotland*

Average lunchtime intake of:	Paid school meal	Free school meal	Paid school meal most days	Free school meal most days	Home	Packed lunch
Energy kJ	2,270	2,370	2,370	(2,030)	2,170	2,550
Per cent of daily energy intake (5 day)	31	31	31	(27)	29	31
Protein g	16.7	17.1	16.4	(14.6)	15.6	15.5
Fat g	26.0	26.4	26.0	(21.4)	22.6	26.9
Fat as per cent of energy	42	41	41	(39)	39	39
Carbohydrate g	63	68	71	(61)	67	80
Calcium mg	140	230	190	(190)	220	210
Iron mg	2.5	2.5	2.4	(2.3)	2.6	2.8
Retinol µg	50	80	60	(50)	150	110
Carotene µg	300	410	290	(240)	270	150
Retinol equivalent µg	100	150	100	(100)	190	140
Thiamin mg	0.21	0.22	0.21	(0.19)	0.24	0.29
Riboflavin mg	0.27	0.34	0.28	(0.27)	0.31	0.24
Nicotinic acid mg	2.8	2.9	2.9	(2.5)	2.6	3.0
Nicotinic acid equivalent mg	6.3	6.4	6.2	(5.5)	5.9	6.1
Vitamin C mg	10.3	10.4	10.3	(10.0)	8.2	21.5
Vitamin D µg	0.13	0.18	0.19	(0.18)	0.38	0.67
Pyridoxine mg	0.28	0.29	0.29	(0.24)	0.24	0.27
Base	54	63	37	(19)	166	65

Table 32: Average daily nutrient intakes of children aged 10/11 years according to type of school meal (excluding those not taking a school meal)

Average daily intake of:	Boys			Girls		
	Cafeteria	Fixed price	Other	Cafeteria	Fixed price	Other
Energy kJ	8,800	8,610	9,070	8,090	7,700	7,240
Protein g	61.3	60.8	62.7	54.3	53.4	49.8
Fat g	88.6	87.1	91.5	84.6	80.6	73.2
Carbohydrate g	279	272	283	251	242	230
Calcium mg	830	820	920	670	710	660
Iron mg	10.0	10.0	10.4	9.1	8.6	7.9
Retinol µg	480	610	560	440	450	650
Carotene µg	1,420	1,540	1,640	1,610	1,390	1,110
Retinol equivalent µg	710	870	830	710	680	830
Thiamin mg	1.25	1.20	1.26	1.01	1.04	0.95
Riboflavin mg	1.74	1.69	1.79	1.33	1.41	1.34
Nicotinic acid mg	15.1	14.6	15.0	13.0	12.7	12.0
Nicotinic acid equivalent mg	26.8	26.4	27.2	23.8	23.1	21.7
Vitamin C mg	65.7	47.3	51.6	64.4	48.3	42.7
Vitamin D µg	1.32	1.49	1.54	1.43	1.32	1.20
Pyridoxine mg	1.16	1.17	1.19	1.04	1.04	0.96
Height cm (s.d)	145.5(5.3)	142.6(6.3)	141.1(5.9)	142.3(4.9)	142.3(7.8)	141.2(5.0)
Base (weighted)	47	418	25	25	388	23

Table 33: *Average daily nutrient intakes of children aged 14/15 years according to type of school meal (excluding those not taking a school meal)*

Average daily intake of:	Boys			Girls		
	Cafeteria	Fixed price	Other	Cafeteria	Fixed price	Other
Energy kJ	10,380	10,450	(10,720)	7,860	7,800	*
Protein g	74.2	76.5	(78.0)	56.4	55.3	*
Fat g	105.9	107.8	(108.1)	82.5	80.6	*
Carbohydrate g	324	321	(336)	240	242	*
Calcium mg	930	920	(860)	690	670	*
Iron mg	12.1	12.5	(12.1)	9.3	8.9	*
Retinol µg	710	650	(380)	560	540	*
Carotene µg	1,670	1,570	(1,100)	1,470	1,330	*
Retinol equivalent µg	990	910	(570)	810	760	*
Thiamin mg	1.47	1.45	(1.43)	1.05	0.49	*
Riboflavin mg	1.90	1.89	(1.70)	1.33	1.24	*
Nicotinic acid mg	18.3	18.3	(16.8)	13.0	12.3	*
Nicotinic acid equivalent mg	32.5	23.1	(32.0)	24.1	23.1	*
Vitamin C mg	50.0	46.0	(43.2)	48.9	44.7	*
Vitamin D µg	1.62	1.60	(2.34)	1.24	1.16	*
Pyridoxine mg	1.34	1.38	(1.35)	1.08	1.00	*
Height cm (s.d)	166.5(8.0)	163.9(10.1)	169.4(6.9)	160.2(6.5)	159.5(7.9)	*
Base	182	30	(4)	162	22	*

74

Table 34: *Foods consumed by boys aged 10/11 years (g/head/week)**

| Food | National median | | Social class (excludes unemployed and one parent families) | | | | | |
		I	II	IIInm	IIIm	IV	V
Number of children	902	48	220	84	219	76	30
Cereals:							
White bread	429(469)	366(354)	419(412)	369(394)	478(559)	476(515)	338(403)
Brown bread	0(123)	0(229)	0(90)	0(50)	0(120)	0(97)	0(170)
	149	22	35	13	30	9	5
Whole meal bread	0(200)	42(99)	0(207)	0(255)	0(58)	0(286)	0(59)
	222		84	24	29	12	5
Other bread	0(127)	0(37)	0(122)	0(111)	0(117)	0(142)	0(146)
	266	23	90	16	54	21	7
Total bread	(579)	(574)	(556)	(495)	(625)	(611)	(475)
Bran products	0(139)	0(0)	0(187)	0(94)	0(55)	0(149)	0(0)
	33	0	17	5	3	3	0
Buns and pastries	43(69)	0(86)	55(83)	48(76)	42(66)	30(61)	40(59)
		17					
Cakes	136(167)	149(202)	169(195)	100(130)	139(164)	120(176)	174(177)
Biscuits	179(203)	142(160)	213(233)	170(202)	158(199)	179(192)	190(204)
Breakfast cereals	225(245)	259(317)	231(257)	237(251)	196(220)	186(237)	199(212)
Puddings, etc	379(428)	356(397)	363(411)	396(453)	364(410)	453(478)	393(391)
Icecream	35(67)	44(76)	68(86)	46(67)	31(52)	24(54)	0(316)
							11
Rice	0(185)	0(179)	0(161)	0(244)	0(140)	0(291)	0(249)
	224	16	70	26	39	11	5
Pasta	0(205)	0(209)	0(221)	56(95)	0(218)	0(155)	84(197)
	427	21	97		94	35	

***Median with mean in brackets, number consuming food below mean (see para 9.1 and Appendix A, para 6.2)**

75

Table 34 (Cont)

Food	National median	Social class (excludes unemployed and one parent families)					
		I	II	IIInm	IIIm	IV	V
Milk and milk products:							
Cows milk, whole	1,710(1,868)	2,442(2,276)	1,886(2,142)	1,632(1,667)	1,642(1,814)	1,755(1,860)	1,667(1,826)
Skimmed, semi skimmed milk	0(900) 27	0(670) 1	0(730) 12	0(0) 0	0(684) 6	0(1,249) 1	0(0) 0
Other milk	0(62) 156	0(44) 7	0(64) 26	0(26) 10	0(45) 39	0(109) 12	0(60) 8
Yogurt	0(247) 323	0(298) 18	14(128)	0(397) 22	0(234) 71	0(267) 25	0(277) 11
Cream	0(26) 282	0(19) 18	0(30) 92	0(23) 24	0(28) 52	0(27) 18	0(18) 11
Cottage cheese	0(20) 6	0(0) 0	0(15) 4	0(0) 0	0(40) 1	0(0) 0	0(0) 0
Cheese	51(86)	69(104)	67(102)	39(64)	60(88)	44(80)	42(63)
Eggs, egg dishes	103(127)	80(127)	103(124)	96(136)	90(116)	126(128)	80(99)
Fats and oils:							
Butter	20(42)	21(29)	20(46)	35(45)	24(47)	10(44)	14(34)
Margarine	9(39)	26(64)	12(39)	0(49)	3(39)	11(47)	4(33)
Low fat spread	0(89) 14	0(0) 0	0(110) 3	0(310) 31	0(95) 6	0(13) 2	0(0) 0
Vegetable oils	0(9) 15	0(5) 6	0(0) 0	0(0) 0	0(14) 3	0(0) 0	0(0) 0
Other fats & oils	0(44) 40	0(7) 3	0(1) 13	0(106) 8	0(33) 7	0(93) 5	0(0) 0

Table 34 (Cont)

Food		Social class (excludes unemployed and one parent families)					
	National median	I	II	IIInm	IIIm	IV	V
Carcase meats:							
Bacon and ham	29(50)	53(79)	36(55)	24(46)	30(51)	37(51)	16(36)
Beef and veal	42(87)	70(91)	27(87)	50(82)	51(98)	41(85)	0(161) 11
Mutton and lamb	0(114) 316	0(85) 22	0(85) 64	0(72) 29	0(113) 86	0(135) 17	0(93) 8
Pork	0(88) 386	0(139) 23	0(67) 85	0(95) 35	0(85) 102	0(81) 27	44(44)
Other meat:							
Chicken fried in breadcrumbs	0(105) 17	0(0) 0	0(117) 5	0(0) 0	0(63) 4	0(139) 76	0(0) 0
Poultry and game	60(88)	105(121)	72(85)	3(126)	56(73)	44(83)	40(73)
Liver	190	0(74) 15	0(86) 46	0(119) 32	0(16) 42	0(75) 15	0(158) 3
Kidney	0(24) 6	0(0) 0	0(0) 0	0(0) 0	0(28) 2	0(27) 2	0(0) 0
Other offals	0(67) 39	0(10) 3	0(109) 9	0(49) 4	0(45) 9	0(168) 2	0(0) 0
Sausages	88(113)	92(101)	90(107)	70(103)	90(114)	87(103)	74(117)
Burgers	18(46)	40(46)	25(40)	0(84) 33	36(50)	0(92) 36	0(107) 9
Other meat products	320(364)	272(259)	346(349)	321(338)	316(402)	304(330)	399(513)

Table 34 (Cont)

Food	National median	Social class (excludes unemployed and one parent families)					
		I	II	IIInm	IIIm	IV	V
Fish and fish products:							
Fish in batter or breadcrumbs	0(138) 325	0(179) 20	0(135) 93	0(161) 38	0(109) 65	0(120) 25	0(69) 7
Fish fingers	0(95) 379	0(128) 23	0(85) 84	0(113) 32	0(85) 96	1(54)	0(93) 14
Shell fish	0(34) 22	0(0) 0	0(16) 2	0(0) 0	0(30) 12	0(18) 1	0(0) 0
Other fish	0(84) 330	48(54)	0(80) 83	34(55)	0(80) 75	0(167) 18	0(71) 10
Sugar, sweets:							
Sugar	112(138)	45(70)	91(121)	60(104)	120(139)	120(154)	189(188)
Syrup and preserves	14(33)	24(44)	30(38)	0(69) 40	15(35)	10(32)	0(64) 13
Chocolate	78(119)	84(126)	88(128)	84(110)	86(134)	51(75)	32(58)
Sweets	59(101)	44(57)	52(83)	40(62)	57(90)	66(150)	78(121)
Potatoes and potato products:							
Crisps, corn snacks, etc	95(104)	65(72)	106(116)	124(120)	111(116)	77(99)	49(91)
Chips	404(441)	188(269)	386(354)	300(416)	404(446)	352(400)	538(545)
Potatoes	483(509)	496(508)	436(457)	466(478)	480(555)	428(464)	566(557)

Table 34 (Cont)

Food	National median	Social class (excludes unemployed and one parent families)					
		I	II	IIInm	IIIm	IV	V
Vegetables:							
Carrots	30(51)	28(48)	37(56)	35(38)	28(52)	45(53)	20(63)
Tomatoes	0(95) 426	46(63)	26(61)	11(29) 31	0(88) 99	0(83) 27	0(77) 12
Baked beans	116(160)	202(235)	86(141)	108(126)	96(145)	154(181)	206(192)
Peas	66(90)	88(68)	33(58)	118(112)	76(105)	48(84)	118(141)
Salad vegetables	0(51) 429	31(41)	10(29)	0(64)	4(27)	0(44) 35	0(38) 14
Other vegetables	119(152)	153(181)	135(172)	129(167)	105(147)	83(126)	84(159)
Fruit:							
Citrus fruit	0(195) 319	0(207) 15	0(190) 97	0(222) 32	0(179) 73	0(189) 25	0(191) 57
Apples and pears	104(163)	143(233)	122(173)	82(167)	120(152)	109(160)	0(329) 10
Other fresh fruit	0(169) 379	42(104)	0(193) 101	0(125) 28	0(140) 101	0(188) 32	0(228) 7
Other fruit	0(108) 448	25(78)	6(53)	0(99) 37	4(50)	4(56)	0(125) 47
Nuts:							
Nuts	0(32) 124	0(31) 7	0(31) 37	0(16) 17	0(42) 30	0(20) 9	0(0) 0
Peanut butter	0(44) 64	0(21) 3	0(38) 22	0(27) 7	0(54) 12	0(32) 3	0(0) 0

Table 34 (Cont)

Food	National median	Social class (excludes unemployed and one parent families)					
		I	II	IIInm	IIIm	IV	V
Beverages:							
Fruit juices	0(450)	176(294)	119(275)	0(462)	0(402)	0(373)	0(765)
	322			22	58	18	3
Tea	731(1,098)	709(1,056)	659(1,034)	400(718)	927(1,133)	672(1,082)	2,014(1,502)
Coffee	0(29)	0(25)	0(38)	0(31)	0(10)	0(60)	1(22)
	384	23	99	26	101	32	
Cocoa, drinking chocolate, etc	0(21)	0(19)	0(17)	0(17)	0(26)	0(31)	0(11)
	157	7	44	9	44	10	5
Horlicks, Ovaltine	0(29)	0(34)	0(26)	0(43)	0(25)	0(23)	0(18)
	201	1	29	21	43	18	13
Milk shakes	0(310)	0(0)	0(317)	0(0)	0(296)	0(0)	0(0)
	12	0	8	0	4	0	0
Colas	0(540)	0(349)	0(611)	0(441)	0(551)	0(493)	0(492)
	387	16	108	39	105	31	13
Fizzy drinks	492(741)	400(772)	528(824)	598(721)	565(789)	542(760)	218(470)
Other soft drinks	51(186)	202(240)	114(230)	136(253)	40(151)	31(166)	70(153)
Alcoholic drinks:							
Beers and lagers	0(154)	0(0)	0(235)	0(174)	0(86)	0(234)	0(0)
	25	0	4	3	7	1	0
Wines	0(64)	0(44)	0(49)	0(54)	0(114)	0(89)	0(0)
	35	5	14	6	5	3	0
Spirits	0(0)	0(0)	0(0)	0(0)	0(0)	0(0)	0(0)
	0	0	0	0	0	0	0

Table 34 (Cont)

Food	Social class (excludes unemployed and one parent families)						
	National median	I	II	IIInm	IIIm	IV	V
Other foods:							
Pickles and sauces	18(38)	29(40)	27(50)	28(41)	12(36)	10(30)	0(52) 15
Soups	0(344) 332	0(329) 22	0(353) 85	0(326) 30	0(315) 76	0(396) 22	0(343) 9
Number of children	902	48	220	84	219	76	30

Table 35: *Foods consumed by boys aged 10/11 years (g/head/week)*

Food	Total Scotland sample	Region London and SE	North	Rest of GB
Number of children	457	238	260	317
Cereals:				
White bread	451(496)	398(437)	427(464)	445(489)
Brown bread	0(91)	0(94)	0(158)	0(116)
	13	35	51	50
Wholemeal bread	0(173)	0(177)	0(195)	0(240)
	17	72	68	65
Other bread	0(127)	0(137)	0(135)	0(116)
	12	67	69	117
Total bread	(564)	(544)	(581)	(599)
Bran products	0(202)	0(43)	0(121)	0(170)
	4	4	13	12
Buns and pastries	39(64)	40(61)	52(82)	40(67)
Cakes	98(121)	160(189)	124(159)	147(169)
Biscuits	129(159)	204(228)	172(200)	172(199)
Breakfast cereals	192(221)	235(268)	232(235)	210(244)
Puddings, etc	285(354)	338(398)	448(500)	382(410)
Icecream	39(64)	34(62)	48(75)	27(64)
Rice	0(169)	0(231)	0(163)	0(163)
	17	73	71	63
Pasta	37(107)	62(120)	0(184)	0(217)
			108	134

Table 35 (Cont)

Food	Region			
	Total Scotland sample	London and SE	North	Rest of GB
Milk and milk products:				
Cows milk, whole	2,061(2,127)	1,756(1,925)	1,642(1,851)	1,690(1,771)
Skimmed, semi-skimmed milk	0(1,136)	0(474)	0(1,015)	0(1,186)
	5	9	6	7
Other milk	0(29)	0(69)	0(69)	0(63)
	20	46	57	33
Yogurt	0(257)	0(259)	0(256)	0(227)
	23	88	100	111
Cream	0(27)	0(28)	0(22)	0(28)
	23	90	73	97
Cottage cheese	0(0)	0(0)	0(0)	0(17)
	0	0	0	6
Cheese	66(111)	57(96)	22(65)	57(90)
Eggs, egg dishes	106(133)	83(103)	112(141)	104(133)
Fats and oils:				
Butter	20(42)	20(44)	10(36)	25(46)
Margarine	10(31)	0(62)	19(45)	8(44)
	2	116	8	5
Low fat spread	0(30)	0(0)	0(100)	0(92)
	2	0	8	5
Vegetable oils	0(8)	0(8)	0(18)	0(8)
	2	7	1	5
Other fats and oils	0(41)	0(34)	0(17)	0(81)
	3	15	10	11

Table 35 (Cont)

Food	Region			
	Total Scotland sample	London and SE	North	Rest of GB
Carcase meats:				
Bacon and ham	40(60)	30(46)	27(47)	30(52)
Beef and veal	127(165)	0(161) 117	55(82)	18(78)
Mutton and lamb	0(88) 18	0(106) 94	0(129) 111	0(110) 94
Pork	0(86) 28	0(95) 107	0(81) 105	0(88) 146
Other meat:				
Chicken fried in breadcrumbs	0(117) 2	0(106) 11	0(0) 0	0(101) 3
Poultry and game	32(78)	72(98)	46(83)	62(86)
Liver	0(89) 13	0(75) 49	0(84) 41	0(104) 87
Kidney	0(0) 0	0(0) 0	0(24) 4	0(24) 2
Other offals	0(81) 8	0(10) 3	0(54) 17	0(93) 11
Sausages	124(146)	88(103)	90(119)	79(108)
Burgers	0(108) 39	46(67)	20(45)	0(73) 131
Other meat products	203(247)	298(349)	327(395)	351(380)

Table 35 (Cont)

Food	Region			
	Total Scotland sample	London and SE	North	Rest of GB
Fish and fish products:				
Fish in batter or breadcrumbs	0(132)	0(144)	0(140)	0(132)
	38	64	110	113
Fish fingers	0(89)	0(94)	0(107)	0(85)
	25	101	125	129
Shellfish	0(65)	0(41)	0(34)	0(17)
	1	7	8	5
Other fish	0(87)	0(76)	0(82)	0(90)
	17	80	100	134
Sugar, sweets:				
Sugar	104(130)	112(147)	116(146)	109(128)
Syrup and preserves	13(35)	24(38)	10(30)	14(32)
Chocolate	105(133)	80(144)	56(101)	80(117)
Sweets	101(142)	60(93)	68(120)	43(80)
Potatoes and potato products:				
Crisps, corn snacks, etc	100(117)	89(113)	68(91)	106(106)
Chips	390(438)	390(386)	460(518)	388(419)
Potatoes	430(453)	478(505)	410(423)	575(597)

Table 35 (Cont)

Food		Region		
	Total Scotland sample	London and SE	North	Rest of GB
Vegetables:				
Carrots	0(57)	25(47)	44(53)	40(61)
	31			
Tomatoes	0(78)	0(96)	0(88)	19(57)
	30	106	109	
Baked beans	96(133)	140(187)	108(155)	112(150)
Peas	28(45)	58(82)	88(98)	76(103)
Salad vegetables	0(47)	0(47)	0(40)	8(33)
	30	114	116	
Other vegetables	68(109)	148(203)	110(134)	148(172)
Fruit:				
Citrus fruit	0(229)	0(208)	0(162)	0(205)
	29	79	93	118
Apples and pears	118(173)	108(159)	62(154)	115(170)
Other fresh fruit	0(165)	0(153)	0(163)	0(182)
	36	82	110	151
Other fruit	34(67)	0(109)	4(49)	4(57)
		108		
Nuts:				
Nuts	0(25)	0(43)	0(35)	0(22)
	9	35	37	43
Peanut butter	0(61)	0(51)	0(49)	0(33)
	6	28	3	28

Table 35 (Cont)

Food	Region			
	Total Scotland sample	London and SE	North	Rest of GB
Beverages:				
Fruit juices	0(557) 23	0(509) 119	0(520) 63	0(332) 117
Tea	827(1,162)	832(1,005)	696(1,036)	676(1,201)
Coffee	0(35) 24	0(50) 86	0(19) 130	0(25) 143
Cocoa, drinking chocolate, etc	0(17) 11	0(17) 43	0(19) 40	0(26) 62
Horlicks, Ovaltine	0(39) 24	0(21) 50	0(36) 79	0(22) 48
Milk shakes	0(0) 0	0(280) 2	0(300) 3	0(330) 5
Colas	156(337)	0(579) 112	0(465) 92	0(536) 137
Fizzy drinks	438(722)	416(651)	576(812)	530(754)
Other soft drinks	102(278)	86(200)	47(155)	40(175)
Alcoholic drinks:				
Beers and Lagers	0(0) 0	0(89) 7	0(144) 5	0(193) 11
Wines	0(0) 0	0(68) 11	0(119) 3	0(59) 21
Spirits	0(0) 0	0(0) 0	0(0) 0	0(0) 0

Table 35 (Cont)

Food	Total Scotland sample	Region		
		London and SE	North	Rest of GB
Other foods:				
Pickles and sauces	0(50) 39	22(50)	16(26)	24(43)
Soups	360(431)	0(279) 68	0(254) 97	0(343) 102
Number of children	457	238	260	317

Table 36: *Foods consumed by boys aged 10/11 years (g/head/week)*

	Family composition						
	One parent families			Two parent families			
Food	One child	Two or more children	All one parent families	One child	Two children	Three children	Four or more children
Number of children	34	71	105	91	447	188	73
Cereals:							
White bread	273(431)	396(450)	384(443)	457(523)	431(462)	407(463)	468(494)
Brown bread	0(63)	0(124)	0(107)	0(111)	0(121)	0(145)	0(100)
	4	16	22	8	82	30	10
Wholemeal bread	0(312)	0(93)	0(179)	0(223)	0(173)	0(250)	0(313)
	12	17	30	17	125	36	16
Other bread	0(185)	0(93)	0(116)	0(140)	0(116)	0(111)	0(224)
	6	14	21	17	136	67	25
Total bread	(581)	(520)	(539)	(602)	(567)	(574)	(652)
Bran products	0(140)	0(37)	0(78)	0(94)	0(149)	0(224)	0(125)
	1	2	3	3	23	1	3
Buns and pastries	53(65)	20(58)	42(62)	0(103)	46(75)	44(68)	48(80)
				41			
Cakes	60(138)	46(130)	101(132)	140(186)	150(176)	150(167)	108(140)
Biscuits	140(142)	143(199)	143(182)	183(199)	192(212)	156(193)	181(216)
Breakfast cereals	216(220)	206(217)	186(214)	117(168)	224(255)	281(269)	283(265)
Puddings, etc	332(470)	370(465)	350(467)	278(333)	410(436)	378(434)	391(423)
Icecream	0(200)	50(70)	0(133)	19(39)	48(82)	30(50)	23(47)
	13		56				
Rice	0(247)	0(141)	0(170)	0(265)	0(171)	0(172)	0(243)
	8	22	30	26	112	45	11
Pasta	56(94)	90(125)	72(112)	0(260)	0(207)	0(184)	0(223)
				41	211	72	29

89

Table 36 (Cont)

Food	Family composition						
	One parent families			Two parent families			
	One child	Two or more children	All one parent families	One child	Two children	Three children	Four or more children
Milk and milk products:							
Cows milk, whole	1,552(1,710)	1,436(1,736)	1,436(1,718)	1,469(1,651)	1,763(1,905)	1,836(2,007)	1,785(1,754)
Skimmed, semi skimmed milk	0(526) / 2	0(1,285) / 3	0(986) / 5	0(1,640) / 1	0(813) / 19	0(1,221) / 1	0(0) / 0
Other milk	0(82) / 9	0(26) / 11	0(52) / 21	0(57) / 9	0(82) / 75	0(47) / 36	0(18) / 14
Yogurt	0(256) / 9	0(166) / 23	0(192) / 33	0(249) / 35	0(105) / 61	0(262) / 61	0(148) / 12
Cream	0(33) / 13	0(18) / 23	0(24) / 37	0(35) / 18	0(28) / 143	0(24) / 61	0(18) / 25
Cottage cheese	0(14) / 1	0(0) / 0	0(16) / 1	0(0) / 0	0(21) / 5	0(0) / 0	0(0) / 0
Cheese	20(66)	39(83)	32(77)	35(79)	67(98)	41(74)	24(64)
Eggs, egg dishes	50(93)	104(128)	95(116)	123(139)	96(114)	134(151)	114(147)
Fats and oils:							
Butter	10(37)	19(37)	17(38)	21(47)	20(41)	28(50)	12(35)
Margarine	19(38)	17(35)	17(35)	2(33)	5(39)	9(39)	24(53)
Low fat spread	0(0) / 0	0(59) / 2	0(59) / 2	0(0) / 0	0(94) / 9	0(0) / 0	0(96) / 3
Vegetable oils	0(10) / 2	0(0) / 0	0(10) / 3	0(16) / 1	0(7) / 6	0(8) / 5	0(0) / 0
Other fats and oils	0(15) / 2	0(0) / 0	0(19) / 2	0(22) / 1	0(64) / 19	0(26) / 18	0(0) / 0

Table 36 (Cont)

				Family composition			
	One parent families			Two parent families			
Food	One child	Two or more children	All one parent families	One child	Two children	Three children	Four or more children
Carcase meats:							
Bacon and ham	23(44)	22(48)	23(47)	33(47)	35(57)	21(41)	20(36)
Beef and veal	0(244)	0(162)	0(190)	48(83)	50(91)	0(173)	35(75)
	17	31	50			93	
Mutton and lamb	20(76)	0(124)	0(135)	0(79)	0(102)	0(134)	0(150)
		19	37	29	161	65	24
Pork	0(120)	0(91)	0(100)	10(44)	0(84)	0(87)	0(96)
	13	26	40		191	79	30
Other meat:							
Chicken fried in breadcrumbs	0(0)	0(111)	0(111)	0(111)	0(91)	0(139)	0(0)
	0	5	5	2	8	2	0
Poultry and game	20(117)	62(82)	53(94)	60(91)	56(82)	77(90)	42(105)
Liver	0(198)	0(109)	0(124)	0(103)	0(102)	0(57)	0(96)
	4	17	21	11	94	55	10
Kidney	0(0)	0(0)	0(0)	0(0)	0(22)	0(34)	0(20)
	0	0	0	0	3	1	2
Other offals	0(21)	0(67)	0(55)	0(153)	0(67)	0(40)	0(121)
	1	4	5	2	16	12	5
Sausages	130(170)	90(107)	90(125)	82(114)	85(112)	90(118)	70(90)
Burgers	0(122)	40(65)	35(61)	40(47)	0(88)	0(95)	0(68)
	16				224	91	34
Other meat products	364(384)	284(337)	306(347)	262(343)	322(364)	280(335)	408(477)

Table 36 (Cont)

	Family composition						
	One parent families			Two parent families			
Food	One child	Two or more children	All one parent families	One child	Two children	Three children	Four or more children
Fish and fish products:							
Fish in batter or breadcrumbs	0(172) 14	0(132) 24	0(146) 38	0(155) 40	0(126) 159	0(163) 64	0(100) 25
Fish fingers	0(128) 10	0(101) 28	0(105) 39	0(93) 39	0(97) 177	0(46) 37	0(92) 27
Shellfish	0(0) 0	0(36) 4	0(36) 4	0(39) 2	0(34) 7	0(39) 6	0(15) 2
Other fish	0(68) 5	0(68) 15	0(68) 21	0(78) 39	0(88) 179	0(85) 67	0(76) 25
Sugar, sweets:							
Sugar	141(191)	144(167)	141(172)	103(134)	95(124)	114(136)	187(186)
Syrup and preserves	15(47)	7(19)	8(27)	0(54) 45	16(36)	17(32)	15(32)
Chocolate	102(160)	68(120)	80(136)	68(129)	85(123)	70(98)	66(119)
Sweets	115(140)	85(130)	104(136)	36(84)	50(96)	70(104)	60(99)
Potatoes and potato products:							
Crisps, corn snacks, etc	42(78)	75(82)	65(83)	124(139)	103(111)	75(95)	52(75)
Chips	464(514)	520(570)	518(550)	464(524)	376(399)	388(414)	443(504)
Potatoes	577(584)	561(554)	546(554)	553(507)	453(490)	457(494)	581(593)

Table 36 (Cont)

	Family composition						
	One parent families			Two parent families			
Food	One child	Two or more children	All one parent families	One child	Two children	Three children	Four or more children
Vegetables:							
Carrots	2(40)	0(71) 31	0(71) 50	27(45)	36(53)	25(46)	51(82)
Tomatoes	0(106) 13	4(47)	0(97) 47	0(86) 38	8(50)	0(104) 81	0(54) 32
Baked beans	112(176)	208(195)	150(188)	138(182)	112(162)	110(138)	96(130)
Peas	56(94)	55(102)	55(97)	90(102)	74(87)	61(86)	60(93)
Salad vegetables	0(56) 16	0(43) 28	0(47) 45	14(29)	0(57) 211	0(44) 91	0(37) 29
Other vegetables	60(148)	151(159)	124(152)	86(151)	129(170)	112(146)	101(191)
Fruit:							
Citrus fruit	0(294) 15	0(183) 30	0(220) 45	0(134) 31	0(99) 147	0(191) 69	0(217) 27
Apples and pears	11(156)	0(323) 30	0(306) 50	82(134)	114(175)	90(161)	120(159)
Other fresh fruit	0(214) 14	0(229) 23	0(223) 37	0(197) 37	0(159) 198	0(162) 79	0(160) 28
Other fruit	13(75)	3(63)	5(66)	0(108) 36	0(115) 217	15(53)	0(77) 36
Nuts:							
Nuts	0(56) 4	0(31) 8	0(40) 12	0(25) 12	0(33) 67	0(33) 21	0(30) 12
Peanut butter	0(42) 7	0(20) 1	0(39) 8	0(49) 4	0(58) 31	0(39) 17	0(104) 5

Table 36 (Cont)

	Family composition						
	One parent families			Two parent families			
Food	One child	Two or more children	All one parent families	One child	Two children	Three children	Four or more children
Beverages:							
Fruit juices	6(273)	0(443) 20	0(446) 41	0(587) 31	0(449) 179	0(446) 59	0(94) 15
Tea	943(1,177)	1,000(1,332)	943(1,266)	542(922)	708(1,442)	910(1,126)	1,000(1,560)
Coffee	0(13) 13	0(32) 20	0(24) 35	0(8) 34	0(36) 195	0(28) 84	1(11)
Cocoa, drinking chocolate, etc.	0(8) 1	0(20) 13	0(19) 15	0(23) 14	0(22) 77	0(21) 37	0(13) 15
Horlicks, Ovaltine	0(25) 7	0(34) 20	0(32) 29	0(24) 22	0(29) 81	0(29) 50	0(33) 19
Milk shakes	0(0) 0	0(0) 0	0(0) 0	0(0) 0	0(307) 5	0(322) 6	0(0) 0
Colas	0(474) 14	0(496) 31	0(500) 46	180(395)	0(551) 203	0(432) 67	0(409) 24
Fizzy drinks	570(715) 11	415(613)	484(683)	492(745)	598(811)	480(700)	296(539)
Other soft drinks	0(435) 11	0(273) 30	0(317) 41	50(206)	110(223)	70(149)	0(257) 31

Table 36 (Cont)

| | Family composition | | | | | | |
| | One parent families | | | Two parent families | | | |
Food	One child	Two or more children	All one parent families	One child	Two children	Three children	Four or more children
Alcoholic drinks:							
Beers and lagers	0(0) 0	0(142) 3	0(142) 3	0(86) 4	0(243) 8	0(115) 10	0(0) 0
Wines	0(40) 1	0(0) 0	0(49) 2	0(0) 0	0(69) 22	0(57) 11	0(0) 0
Spirits	0(0) 0	0(0) 0	0(0) 0	0(0) 0	0(0) 0	0(0) 0	0(0) 0
Other foods:							
Pickles and sauces	10(59)	17(31)	14(39)	4(32)	21(43)	20(33)	18(27)
Soups	0(251) 8	0(306) 25	0(299) 33	0(347) 42	0(333) 178	0(353) 57	0(482) 22
Number of children	34	71	105	91	447	188	73

Table 37: *Foods consumed by boys aged 10/11 years (g/head/week)*

Food	Employment and benefits (benefits are also received by one parent families)				
	Father unemployed	Father in employment	Family Income Supplement (FIS)	Supplementary Benefit (SB)	Neither FIS or SB
Number of children	123	677	32	135	728
Cereals:					
White bread	432(501)	430(464)	447(501)	432(514)	427(458)
Brown bread	0(124) 16	0(124) 115	0(0) 0	0(168) 17	0(117) 132
Wholemeal bread	0(234) 9	0(201) 182	0(251) 10	0(177) 17	0(200) 195
Other bread	0(217) 34	0(114) 210	0(71) 13	0(213) 40	0(114) 212
Total bread	(594)	(574)	(608)	(618)	(566)
Bran products	0(40) 1	0(148) 29	0(0) 0	0(0) 0	0(140) 32
Buns and pastries	44(71)	43(69)	53(63)	40(65)	43(71)
Cakes	110(137)	150(170)	104(123)	121(152)	145(172)
Biscuits	177(196)	182(105)	191(202)	173(207)	180(203)
Breakfast cereals	251(279)	222(241)	265(266)	246(243)	222(246)
Puddings, etc	398(443)	381(425)	429(418)	404(470)	374(420)
Icecream	0(122) 59	41(68)	30(48)	28(64)	39(69)
Rice	0(200) 31	0(182) 166	0(152) 8	0(185) 40	0(187) 176
Pasta	0(177) 59	0(213) 309	60(110)	38(85)	0(215) 335

Table 37 (Cont)

Food	Employment and benefits (benefits are also received by one parent families)				
	Father unemployed	Father in employment	Family Income Supplement (FIS)	Supplementary Benefit (SB)	Neither FIS or SB
Milk and milk products:					
Cows milk, whole	1,680(1,658)	1,784(1,907)	1,492(1,527)	1,440(1,555)	1,785(1,946)
Skimmed, semi skimmed milk	0(1,872)	0(791)	0(700)	0(1,112)	0(883)
	2	20	3	4	20
Other milk	0(87)	0(57)	0(85)	0(81)	0(56)
	33	102	3	36	117
Yogurt	0(161)	0(265)	0(145)	0(159)	0(262)
	30	257	8	37	277
Cream	0(16)	0(27)	0(14)	0(17)	0(29)
	33	214	9	39	232
Cottage cheese	0(0)	0(22)	0(14)	0(0)	0(21)
	0	5	1	0	5
Cheese	8(68)	55(90)	32(50)	22(74)	57(90)
Eggs, egg dishes	156(164)	101(122)	100(123)	119(135)	102(126)
Fats and oils:					
Butter	10(35)	22(43)	57(77)	11(34)	21(42)
Margarine	20(48)	5(48)	0(71)	23(51)	4(37)
			15		
Low fat spread	0(130)	0(83)	0(0)	0(0)	0(90)
	2	12	0	0	14
Vegetable oils	0(0)	0(8)	0(0)	0(11)	0(8)
	0	12	0	3	12
Other fats and oils	0(11)	0(47)	0(34)	0(11)	0(48)
	2	36	6	2	31

Table 37 (Cont)

Food	Employment and benefits (benefits are also received by one parent families)				
	Father unemployed	Father in employment	Family Income Supplement (FIS)	Supplementary Benefit (SB)	Neither FIS or SB
Carcase meats:					
Bacon and ham	11(32)	32(53)	25(52)	16(40)	30(51)
Beef and veal	35(77)	42(90)	85(112)	0(164) 62	42(88)
Mutton and lamb	0(168) 52	0(98) 226	0(70) 9	0(182) 59	0(100) 248
Pork	0(102) 56	0(84) 290	0(108) 6	0(96) 51	0(86) 327
Other meat:					
Chicken fried in breadcrumbs	0(104) 1	0(102) 11	0(0) 0	0(112) 4	0(102) 12
Poultry and game	34(84)	64(88)	46(80)	32(80)	66(89)
Liver	0(49) 15	0(91) 153	0(93) 11	0(82) 22	0(92) 157
Kidney	0(19) 2	0(28) 4	0(0) 0	0(15) 1	0(27) 5
Other offals	0(63) 8	0(71) 27	0(0) 0	0(56) 9	0(71) 30
Sausages	83(131)	86(110)	88(129)	90(126)	87(110)
Burgers	35(52)	16(45)	40(51)	0(107) 62	22(46)
Other meat products	320(375)	321(362)	335(372)	302(337)	325(369)

Table 37 (Cont)

Food	Employment and benefits (benefits are also received by one parent families)				
	Father unemployed	Father in employment	Family Income Supplement (FIS)	Supplementary Benefit (SB)	Neither FIS or SB
Fish and fish products:					
Fish in batter or breadcrumbs	0(173) 42	0(32) 249	0(95) 5	0(174) 48	0(132) 272
Fish fingers	0(92) 53	0(95) 287	42(46)	0(95) 58	0(96) 301
Shellfish	0(78) 1	0(30) 17	0(0) 0	0(52) 4	0(30) 17
Other fish	0(114) 38	0(82) 265	0(50) 11	0(85) 39	0(82) 277
Sugar, sweets:					
Sugar	166(176)	100(132)	115(165)	156(171)	103(132)
Syrup and preserves	4(24)	17(35)	7(24)	0(43) 67	18(36)
Chocolate	85(122)	79(120)	70(104)	70(117)	79(121)
Sweets	93(132)	50(94)	60(85)	93(149)	50(92)
Potatoes and potato products:					
Crisps, corn snacks, etc	73(86)	100(106)	75(84)	59(80)	98(110)
Chips	544(600)	379(412)	406(440)	552(609)	380(409)
Potatoes	498(527)	468(506)	608(536)	535(541)	468(500)

Table 37 (Cont)

Food	Employment and benefits (benefits are also received by one parent families)				
	Father unemployed	Father in employment	Family Income Supplement (FIS)	Supplementary Benefit (SB)	Neither FIS or SB
Vegetables:					
Carrots	31(55)	35(50)	19(30)	27(52)	32(52)
Tomatoes	0(99) 44	0(93) 331	0(95) 15	0(94) 57	0(95) 350
Baked beans	145(163)	108(157)	210(195)	176(189)	108(153)
Peas	98(118)	66(86)	76(80)	72(98)	64(89)
Salad vegetables	0(42) 38	3(26)	7(19)	0(41) 50	0(54) 359
Other vegetables	84(178)	119(159)	200(170)	95(172)	165(162)
Fruit:					
Citrus fruit	0(200) 30	0(192) 248	69(100)	0(216) 34	0(196) 263
Apples and pears	11(154)	110(165)	87(135)	0(317) 63	112(168)
Other fresh fruit	0(138) 40	0(167) 298	0(187) 14	0(165) 39	0(168) 323
Other fruit	0(96) 53	4(55)	70(53)	0(107) 63	0(111) 360
Nuts:					
Nuts	0(30) 15	0(31) 100	0(38) 5	0(31) 16	0(32) 104
Peanut butter	0(67) 11	0(39) 47	0(67) 1	0(73) 7	0(40) 55

Table 37 (Cont)

Food	Employment and benefits (benefits are also received by one parent families)				
	Father unemployed	Father in employment	Family Income Supplement (FIS)	Supplementary Benefit (SB)	Neither FIS or SB
Beverages:					
Fruit juices	0(207) 27	0(463) 254	0(445) 14	0(217) 29	0(477) 276
Tea	910(1,248)	708(1,068)	972(1,246)	1,248(1,474)	686(1,022)
Coffee	0(31) 58	0(30) 297	0(16) 12	0(36) 57	0(29) 315
Cocoa, drinking chocolate, etc	0(18) 20	0(21) 118	0(8) 2	0(20) 20	0(21) 134
Horlicks, Ovaltine	0(34) 47	0(27) 125	0(25) 2	0(37) 53	0(27) 146
Milk shakes	0(0) 0	0(310) 12	0(0) 0	0(0) 0	0(310) 12
Colas	0(584) 32	0(542) 312	150(211)	0(618) 38	0(542) 329
Fizzy drinks	367(574)	528(760)	580(895)	380(692)	516(738)
Other soft drinks	0(355) 56	75(190)	0(358) 10	0(292) 55	76(200) 55
Alcoholic drinks:					
Beers and lagers	0(268) 3	0(155) 16	0(0) 0	0(309) 2	0(139) 23
Wines	0(138) 1	0(62) 32	0(53) 2	0(0) 0	0(66) 32
Spirits	0(0) 0	0(0) 0	0(0) 0	0(0) 0	0(0) 0

Table 37 (Cont)

Food	Employment and benefits (benefits are also received by one parent families)				
	Father unemployed	Father in employment	Family Income Supplement (FIS)	Supplementary Benefit (SB)	Neither FIS or SB
Other foods:					
Pickles and sauces	3(26)	21(41)	18(33)	12(27)	18(40)
Soups	0(405)	0(339)	0(243)	0(388)	0(339)
	54	244	8	52	273
Number of children	123	677	32	135	728

Table 38: *Food consumed by boys aged 10/11 years (g/head/week)*

Food	Type of lunch						
	Paid school meal	Free school meal	Paid school meal most days	Free school meal most days	Home	Packed lunch	Cafe
Number of children	277	127	97	46	133	256	20
Cereals:							
White bread	310(339)	398(480)	396(440)	378(430)	513(565)	546(557)	576(461)
Brown bread	0(100) 50	0(124) 20	0(68) 5	0(66) 6	0(91) 16	0(155) 46	0(245) 6
Wholemeal bread	0(160) 61	0(151) 14	0(197) 31	0(136) 8	0(330) 17	0(230) 82	0(158) 4
Other bread	0(106) 54	0(273) 33	0(85) 38	0(136) 13	0(185) 29	0(72) 87	27(121) 87
Total bread	(431)	(589)	(539)	(500)	(660)	(685)	(693)
Bran products	0(112) 10	0(0) 0	0(102) 4	0(0) 0	0(67) 8	0(408) 5	0(0) 0
Buns and pastries	67(87)	48(78)	50(70)	45(58)	0(104) 64	0(136) 118	0(80) 8
Cakes	122(169)	131(157)	154(178)	104(124)	100(137)	166(192)	213(193)
Biscuits	187(222)	148(179)	176(206)	134(155)	143(182)	208(224)	163(158)
Breakfast cereals	236(274)	248(261)	214(212)	260(260)	150(179)	231(264)	176(185)
Puddings, etc	532(542)	446(510)	372(409)	429(449)	269(325)	280(360)	208(233)
Icecream	35(74) 59	0(103) 59	41(70)	26(62)	42(67)	44(66)	0(209) 8
Rice	0(215) 65	0(184) 33	0(210) 37	0(184) 9	0(165) 27	0(140) 45	0(160) 7
Pasta	56(108)	90(120)	0(222) 47	0(241) 21	0(307) 58	0(167) 83	0(156) 4

Table 38 (Cont)

Food	Type of lunch						
	Paid school meal	Free school meal	Paid school meal most days	Free school meal most days	Home	Packed lunch	Cafe
Milk and milk products:							
Cow milk, whole	1,846(2,110)	1,440(1,605)	1,628(1,721)	1,611(1,771)	1,658(1,746)	1,770(1,920)	2,234(2,164)
Skimmed, semi skimmed milk	0(650) / 10	0(835) / 3	0(0) / 0	0(200) / 1	0(1,365) / 5	0(982) / 5	0(1,484) / 1
Other milk	0(54) / 54	0(85) / 36	0(60) / 17	0(8) / 10	0(55) / 13	0(92) / 19	0(26) / 4
Yogurt	0(204) / 91	0(166) / 32	0(217) / 41	0(115) / 8	0(229) / 38	0(341) / 99	0(242) / 9
Cream	0(27) / 97	0(14) / 45	0(22) / 35	0(16) / 12	0(29) / 24	0(34) / 64	0(79) / 4
Cottage cheese	0(16) / 1	0(0) / 0	0(0) / 0	0(0) / 0	0(40) / 1	0(15) / 4	0(0) / 0
Cheese	48(85)	26(72)	73(96)	0(117) / 19	39(83)	79(103)	44(60)
Eggs, egg dishes	98(116)	116(152)	120(115)	70(124)	121(141)	92(118)	103(189)
Fats and oils:							
Butter	14(36)	14(34)	26(49)	10(32)	24(43)	20(49)	81(82)
Margarine	3(27)	17(42)	0(51) / 45	22(45)	8(40)	42(56)	0(81) / 6
Low fat spread	0(92) / 5	0(140) / 2	0(12) / 1	0(0) / 0	0(40) / 2	0(121) / 4	0(0) / 0
Vegetable oils	0(0) / 0	0(11) / 3	0(10) / 2	0(0) / 0	0(14) / 2	0(8) / 4	0(5) / 3
Other fats and oils	0(72) / 13	0(0) / 0	0(15) / 4	0(12) / 2	0(35) / 3	0(30) / 17	0(111) / 1

Table 38 (Cont)

Food	Type of lunch						
	Paid school meal	Free school meal	Paid school meal most days	Free school meal most days	Home	Packed lunch	Cafe
Carcase meats:							
Bacon and ham	18(35)	10(31)	57(61)	30(48)	41(62)	45(60)	47(86)
Beef and veal	55(89)	34(86)	18(68)	60(100)	47(86)	0(183) 119	183(115)
Mutton and lamb	0(123) 84	0(166) 59	0(65) 34	0(148) 12	0(123) 31	0(83) 91	0(116) 4
Pork	0(84) 102	0(94) 49	0(73) 45	0(67) 22	0(93) 50	0(95) 99	47(56)
Other meat:							
Chicken fried in breadcrumbs	0(114) 8	0(112) 4	0(0) 0	0(0) 0	0(109) 2	0(28) 2	0(0)
Poultry and game	60(93)	40(86)	70(99)	36(64)	60(79)	72(89)	126(89)
Liver	0(118) 45	0(109) 24	0(80) 18	0(90) 12	0(76) 26	0(77) 50	26(36)
Kidney	0(24) 3	0(15) 1	0(34) 1	0(0) 0	0(0) 0	0(0) 0	0(0) 0
Other offals	0(57) 10	0(61) 8	0(75) 2	0(0) 0	0(79) 7	0(73) 11	0(0) 0
Sausages	85(106)	90(118)	96(120)	88(160)	88(117)	78(102)	99(122)
Burgers	42(56)	39(61)	45(69)	42(49)	0(87) 50	0(77) 98	0(96) 4
Other meat products	360(394)	327(402)	298(340)	247(301)	256(327)	304(356)	440(440)

105

Table 38 (Cont)

Food	Type of lunch						
	Paid school meal	Free school meal	Paid school meal most days	Free school meal most days	Home	Packed lunch	Cafe
Fish and fish products:							
Fish in batter or breadcrumbs	0(142) 92	0(121) 41	0(116) 42	0(90) 18	0(128) 35	0(151) 88	0(290) 7
Fish fingers	48(54) 59	0(92) 59	0(116) 40	41(46) 21	0(96) 44	0(83) 62	63(87) 62
Shellfish	0(42) 5	0(57) 2	0(18) 4	0(0) 0	0(30) 5	0(35) 5	0(0) 0
Other fish	0(98) 81	0(94) 36	0(79) 39	0(76) 16	0(78) 41	0(78) 104	0(39) 8
Sugar, sweets:							
Sugar	87(127)	157(177)	98(133)	166(194)	135(155)	88(115)	113(111)
Syrup and preserves	12(34)	4(25)	18(34)	0(32) 21	12(34)	23(38)	30(52)
Chocolate	74(115)	72(114)	97(123)	77(154)	92(125)	69(10)	135(200)
Sweets	44(92)	88(122)	85(116)	60(125)	68(122)	44(75)	96(132)
Potatoes and potato products:							
Crisps, corn snacks etc	66(96)	54(77)	86(98)	80(91)	100(104)	122(130)	97(120)
Chips	440(490)	514(568)	430(416)	591(638)	408(465)	250(301)	392(437)
Potatoes	490(530)	567(569)	404(438)	511(516)	472(507)	448(488)	445(515)

Table 38 (Cont)

Food	Type of lunch						
	Paid school meal	Free school meal	Paid school meal most days	Free school meal most days	Home	Packed lunch	Cafe
Vegetables:							
Carrots	64(70)	30(52)	20(36)	0(57) 23	15(47)	27(48)	38(43)
Tomatoes	1(47) 60	0(77) 60	20(53)	0(75) 15	0(91) 49	8(54)	0(102) 7
Baked beans	140(184)	172(173)	170(179)	254(252)	106(140)	80(103)	314(351)
Peas	73(103)	72(117)	53(66)	82(98)	64(85)	70(79)	22(52)
Salad vegetables	6(32)	0(38) 54	11(30)	0(52) 15	0(47) 56	0(50) 121	12(20)
Other vegetables	155(192)	164(198)	115(176)	54(122)	94(131)	12(139)	110(141)
Fruit:							
Citrus fruit	0(177) 57	0(195) 44	0(165) 47	0(170) 18	0(233) 50	0(213) 93	0(158) 6
Apples and pears	32(128)	86(174)	80(127)	0(248) 19	109(148)	145(204)	110(207)
Other fresh fruit	0(148) 93	0(163) 45	0(188) 43	0(152) 9	50(105)	0(171) 99	72(127)
Other fruit	6(63)	9(51)	0(115) 45	0(88) 19	0(122) 52	17(52)	45(77)
Nuts:							
Nuts	0(28) 42	0(26) 8	0(21) 8	0(45) 6	0(60) 13	0(28) 42	0(45) 5
Peanut butter	0(38) 16	0(27) 2	0(22) 3	0(54) 2	0(72) 11	0(39) 30	0(0) 0

Table 38 (Cont)

Food	Type of lunch						
	Paid school meal	Free school meal	Paid school meal most days	Free school meal most days	Home	Packed lunch	Cafe
Beverages:							
Fruit juices	0(543) 77	0(289) 28	0(372) 46	0(154) 12	0(498) 33	0(481) 118	0(372) 9
Tea	452(844) 85	995(1,399) 47	540(911) 19	1,156(1,259) 19	1,064(1,292) 59	709(1,106) 104	1,322(1,440) 9
Coffee	0(29) 47	0(22) 27	0(36) 19	0(36) 8	0(18) 59	0(39) 35	3(3) 5
Cocoa, drinking chocolate, etc	0(23) 51	0(16) 27	0(43) 7	0(10) 8	0(22) 23	0(21) 35	0(11) 5
Horlicks, Ovaltine	0(32) 76	0(38) 55	0(20) 24	0(20) 21	0(23) 15	0(12) 9	0(0) 0
Milk shakes	0(330) 1	0(0) 0	0(0) 0	0(0) 0	0(0) 0	0(308) 10	0(0) 0
Colas	0(493) 104	0(506) 34	0(594) 48	0(417) 17	160(344)	0(517) 97	525(410)
Fizzy drinks	565(800)	330(541)	508(733)	510(622)	484(842)	454(736)	646(980)
Other soft drinks	70(150) 53	0(217) 53	131(201) 17	0(354) 17	50(211)	112(259)	33(125)
Alcoholic drinks:							
Beers and lagers	0(111) 15	0(426) 1	0(256) 3	0(0) 0	0(94) 2	0(200) 3	0(0) 0
Wines	0(57) 15	0(0) 0	0(69) 9	0(138) 1	0(28) 2	0(70) 8	0(0) 0
Spirits	0(0) 0	0(0) 0	0(0) 0	0(0) 0	0(0) 0	0(0) 0	0(0) 0

Table 38 (Cont)

Food	Type of lunch						
	Paid school meal	Free school meal	Paid school meal most days	Free school meal most days	Home	Packed lunch	Cafe
Other foods:							
Pickles and sauces	17(34)	14(29)	12(42)	20(34)	14(41)	19(44)	20(39)
Soups	0(320)	0(370)	0(351)	0(272)	146(248)	0(263)	128(154)
	74	48	37	15		73	
Number of children	227	127	97	46	133	256	20

Table 39: *Foods consumed by boys aged 10/11 years (g/head/week)*

Food	Type of school meal (excluding those not taking a school meal)		
	Cafeteria	Fixed price	Other
Number of children	47	418	25
Cereals:			
White bread	351(369)	361(407)	365(402)
Brown bread	0(83)	0(102)	0(0)
	3	78	0
Wholemeal bread	0(192)	0(163)	0(157)
	16	94	4
Other bread	0(58)	0(157)	0(56)
	15	120	4
Total bread	(458)	(507)	(437)
Bran products	0(94)	0(113)	0(0)
	3	11	0
Buns and pastries	42(64)	61(80)	40(80)
Cakes	125(179)	128(160)	146(195)
Biscuits	142(188)	170(201)	224(240)
Breakfast cereals	235(212)	232(262)	248(262)
Puddings, etc	277(348)	472(516)	500(494)
Icecream	40(83)	28(63)	41(77)
Rice	0(122)	0(218)	0(157)
	16	123	5
Pasta	38(86)	60(116)	0(188)
			12
Milk and milk products:			
Cows milk, whole	1,739(1,842)	1,705(1,867)	1,680(2,050)
Skimmed, semi skimmed, milk	0(0)	0(646)	0(0)
	0	15	0
Other milk	0(113)	0(61)	0(20)
	5	102	8
Yogurt	0(171)	0(203)	0(155)
	23	141	8
Cream	4(18)	0(21)	0(15)
		154	11
Cottage cheese	0(0)	0(16)	0(0)
	0	1	0
Cheese	105(102)	42(78)	28(72)
Eggs, egg dishes	120(116)	101(127)	102(118)
Fats and oils:			
Butter	22(39)	14(38)	27(32)
Margarine	8(22)	8(33)	3(32)
Low fat spread	0(0)	0(89)	0(0)
	0	8	0
Vegetable oils	0(0)	0(9)	0(0)
	0	6	0
Other fats and oils	0(10)	0(61)	0(0)
	3	16	0

Table 39 (Cont)

Food	Type of school meal (excluding those not taking a school meal)		
	Cafeteria	Fixed price	Other
Carcase meats:			
Bacon and ham	25(49)	25(40)	0(65)
			11
Beef and veal	20(72)	48(84)	40(125)
Mutton and lamb	0(103)	0(133)	0(42)
	8	171	9
Pork	41(53)	0(81)	0(85)
		181	10
Other meat:			
Chicken fried in breadcrumbs	0(120)	0(101)	0(144)
	4	7	2
Poultry and game	67(77)	54(92)	71(89)
Liver	0(103)	0(107)	0(95)
	7	86	6
Kidney	0(0)	0(24)	0(0)
	0	6	0
Other offals	0(0)	0(60)	0(0)
	0	20	0
Sausages	92(100)	90(117)	110(143)
Burgers	75(93)	40(54)	44(80)
Other meat products	204(303)	344(382)	413(433)
Fish and fish products:			
Fish in batter or breadcrumbs	0(191)	0(123)	0(103)
	11	176	6
Fish fingers	0(128)	20(47)	51(56)
	23		
Shellfish	0(16)	0(33)	0(78)
	2	9	1
Other fish	0(68)	0(94)	0(85)
	17	151	4
Sugar, sweets:			
Sugar	98(120)	122(150)	121(157)
Syrup and preserves	6(29)	10(30)	4(33)
Chocolate	131(178)	68(110)	172(185)
Sweets	36(91)	68(109)	50(122)
Potatoes and potato products:			
Crisps, corn snacks, etc	118(115)	66(89)	75(89)
Chips	474(486)	464(572)	470(504)
Potatoes	496(446)	499(525)	526(587)
Vegetables:			
Carrots	0(71)	44(60)	0(74)
	16		12
Tomotoes	47(57)	0(86)	0(111)
		209	7
Baked beans	190(242)	148(180)	90(192)
Peas	0(122)	72(103)	106(101)
	23		

Table 39 (Cont)

Food	Type of school meal (excluding those not taking a school meal)		
	Cafeteria	Fixed price	Other
Salad vegetables	30(38)	0(55)	0(38)
		193	10
Other vegetables	272(209)	135(181)	190(178)
Fruit:			
Citrus fruit	0(154)	0(184)	0(134)
	21	136	8
Apples and pears	0(259)	75(139)	0(405)
	21		9
Other fresh fruit	0(178)	0(161)	0(120)
	21	160	9
Other fruit	0(113)	6(58)	0(86)
	22		8
Nuts:			
Nuts	0(24)	0(28)	0(33)
	5	54	3
Peanut butter	0(47)	0(29)	0(67)
	7	15	1
Beverages:			
Fruit juices	214(348)	0(420)	0(357)
		119	7
Tea	981(926)	656(1,082)	0(1,106)
			11
Coffee	0(19)	0(30)	4(27)
	20	172	
Cocoa, drinking chocolate, etc	0(47)	0(20)	0(0)
	5	87	0
Horlicks, Ovaltine	0(34)	0(30)	0(34)
	6	158	11
Milk shakes	0(0)	0(330)	0(0)
	0	1	0
Colas	0(549)	0(506)	0(537)
	22	169	12
Fizzy drinks	945(1,009)	438(652)	323(1,015)
Other soft drinks	176(195)	22(137)	39(157)
Alcoholic drinks:			
Beers and lagers	0(0)	0(154)	0(0)
	0	19	0
Wines	0(28)	0(68)	0(0)
	7	4	0
Spirits	0(0)	0(0)	0(0)
	0	0	0
Other foods:			
Pickles and sauces	12(52)	16(31)	17(51)
Soups	0(375)	0(332)	128(168)
	19	141	
Number of children	47	418	25

112

Table 40: *Foods consumed by girls aged 10/11 years (g/head/week)*

Food	National median	Social class (excludes unemployed and one parent families)					
		I	II	IIInm	IIIm	IV	V
Number of children	821	51	182	93	157	70	25
Cereals:							
White bread	381(406) 124	225(220)	301(316)	381(362)	430(465)	468(453)	522(567)
Brown bread	0(118) 124	0(78) 11	0(169) 36	0(83) 19	0(119) 28	0(135) 6	0(96) 2
Wholemeal bread	0(156) 201	0(130) 21	0(201) 64	0(138) 26	0(120) 28	0(200) 12	0(144) 5
Other bread	0(93) 208	0(55) 5	0(75) 64	0(89) 17	0(90) 38	0(100) 16	0(56) 5
Total bread	(485)	(295)	(447)	(434)	(529)	(523)	(616)
Bran products	0(90) 29	0(208) 5	0(39) 9	0(0) 0	0(101) 7	0(108) 2	0(18) 1
Buns and pastries	32(62)	23(108)	46(80)	32(66)	32(53)	0(110) 33	0(132) 12
Cakes	142(173)	142(150)	148(184)	176(174)	148(176)	153(173)	111(144)
Biscuits	160(179)	90(144)	182(198)	137(158)	174(188)	137(189)	183(178)
Breakfast cereals	144(160)	157(161)	186(187)	148(154)	136(162)	100(120)	146(125)
Puddings, etc	334(393)	257(354)	345(404)	370(428)	340(383)	314(353)	168(267)
Icecream	48(72)	35(61)	64(87)	55(72)	50(74)	40(66)	68(71)
Rice	0(148) 193	0(134) 25	0(151) 46	0(406) 11	0(142) 35	0(128) 15	0(88) 4
Pasta	0(193) 397	0(264) 23	50(101)	0(251) 34	0(202) 66	0(160) 31	0(159) 10

Table 40 (Cont)

Food	National median	Social class (excludes unemployed and one parent families)					
		I	II	IIInm	IIIm	IV	V
Milk and milk products:							
Cows milk, whole	1,298(1,401)	1,790(1,737)	1,529(1,578)	1,228(1,601)	1,228(1,446)	1,120(1,206)	1,024(1,180)
Skimmed, semi skimmed milk	0(761)	0(0)	0(275)	0(441)	0(682)	0(2,068)	0(0)
	28	0	8	6	4	1	0
Other milk	0(138)	0(58)	0(42)	0(27)	0(118)	0(113)	0(279)
	31	8	23	5	24	16	7
Yogurt	0(235)	128(184)	0(235)	24(139)	0(238)	0(223)	0(179)
	322		83		54	20	4
Cream	0(27)	0(69)	0(29)	0(26)	0(30)	0(18)	0(19)
	273	16	91	31	36	21	4
Cottage cheese	0(33)	0(0)	0(35)	0(31)	0(0)	0(0)	0(0)
	15	0	4	8	0	0	0
Cheese	50(79)	38(69)	58(91)	35(97)	39(69)	45(78)	54(94)
Eggs, egg dishes	85(113)	101(119)	80(100)	60(95)	82(104)	74(117)	104(156)
Fats and oils:							
Butter	20(38)	18(38)	22(37)	36(48)	31(42)	13(42)	4(22)
Margarine	9(36)	0(40)	4(34)	0(57)	5(37)	6(33)	42(57)
Low fat spread	0(20)	0(2)	0(11)	0(0)	0(39)	0(0)	0(0)
	12	2	3	0	3	0	0
Vegetable oils	0(8)	0(5)	0(9)	0(0)	0(0)	0(0)	0(0)
	13	4	6	0	0	0	0
Other fats and oils	0(41)	0(11)	0(43)	0(0)	0(36)	0(39)	0(0)
	62	4	26	0	5	7	0

114

Table 40 (Cont)

Food		Social class (excludes unemployed and one parent families)					
	National median	I	II	IIInm	IIIm	IV	V
Carcase meats:							
Bacon and ham	35(56)	54(64)	32(51)	28(52)	40(58)	45(81)	0(54) 12
Beef and veal	40(82)	40(84)	64(89)	0(137) 46	44(91)	23(61)	90(130)
Mutton and lamb	0(108) 279	0(136) 10	0(103) 62	28(53)	0(104) 44	0(103) 15	0(115) 7
Pork	0(85) 353	63(54)	0(79) 80	0(75) 39	0(77) 72	0(79) 35	0(77) 6
Other meat:							
Chicken fried in breadcrumbs	0(106) 18	0(0) 0	0(86) 10	0(97) 2	0(170) 4	0(0) 0	0(120) 1
Poultry and game	48(82)	94(111)	56(85)	0(218) 40	44(78)	34(78)	20(101)
Liver	0(64) 153	0(75) 14	0(55) 34	0(88) 26	0(64) 27	0(53) 18	0(64) 9
Kidney	0(54) 9	0(0) 0	0(36) 5	0(0) 0	0(190) 1	0(0) 0	0(0) 0
Other offals	0(95) 27	0(32) 1	0(172) 8	0(0) 0	0(59) 4	0(53) 2	0(0) 0
Sausages	67(85)	110(88)	56(71)	78(72)	76(92)	81(110)	45(83)
Burgers	0(87) 361	0(73) 21	33(58)	0(81) 41	0(89) 69	0(89) 29	0(71) 9
Other meat products	295(322)	295(363)	240(297)	327(337)	270(294)	367(381)	358(364)

115

Table 40 (Cont)

| Food | National median | Social class (excludes unemployed and one parent families) | | | | | |
		I	II	IIInm	IIIm	IV	V
Fish and fish products:							
Fish in batter or breadcrumbs	0(120) 313	0(69) 7	0(111) 80	0(118) 43	0(138) 55	0(107) 31	0(164) 7
Fish fingers	0(83) 326	0(68) 20	0(111) 59	0(100) 32	0(76) 56	0(68) 29	0(54) 11
Shellfish	0(82) 18	0(0) 0	0(23) 4	0(22) 2	0(73) 5	0(188) 5	0(0) 0
Other fish	0(77) 302	0(72) 14	15(36)	0(92) 32	0(74) 43	0(76) 34	0(89) 5
Sugar, sweets:							
Sugar	84(104)	74(89)	67(90)	42(66)	97(106)	116(138)	46(76)
Syrup and preserves	8(27)	20(38)	10(33)	4(26)	16(30)	0(40)	4(16)
Chocolate	72(99)	54(99)	64(81)	84(121)	82(119)	42(103)	44(103)
Sweets	75(116)	88(114)	48(81)	37(76)	60(115)	96(133)	117(145)
Potatoes and potato products:							
Crisps, corn snacks, etc	104(114)	90(89)	102(106)	111(113)	110(126)	128(122)	82(91)
Chips	344(403)	250(240)	246(297)	304(377)	304(416)	393(438)	309(540)
Potatoes	399(422)	360(416)	382(375)	446(425)	432(440)	445(462)	462(461)

Table 40 (Cont)

Food	National median	Social class (excludes unemployed and one parent families)					
		I	II	IIInm	IIIm	IV	V
Vegetables:							
Carrots	31(50)	49(56)	44(56)	30(56)	13(42)	31(44)	14(27)
Tomatoes	7(41)	0(87)	20(49)	0(58)	0(76)	0(74)	0(65)
	19	19		46	70	35	10
Baked beans	90(119)	12(113)	50(76)	92(118)	98(147)	114(125)	60(128)
Peas	60(80)	60(67)	48(69)	80(104)	54(80)	73(82)	42(67)
Salad vegetables	11(32)	34(62)	21(34)	17(35)	6(28)	0(57)	0(28)
						32	11
Other vegetables	129(150)	218(180)	126(146)	128(161)	134(138)	158(158)	143(158)
Fruit:							
Citrus fruit	0(219)	0(186)	77(152)	0(291)	0(152)	0(186)	80(160)
	351	22		93	63	18	
Apples and pears	122(181)	170(222)	126(167)	208(231)	165(212)	148(178)	60(109)
Other fresh fruit	0(160)	88(112)	5(86)	0(190)	0(148)	0(131)	40(78)
	375			43	60	27	
Other fruit	0(122)	23(52)	38(88)	9(74)	0(125)	0(96)	0(118)
	406				67	30	12
Nuts:							
Nuts	0(37)	0(9)	0(41)	0(19)	0(37)	0(72)	0(26)
	89	3	23	5	18	5	2
Peanut butter	0(41)	0(23)	0(42)	0(18)	0(58)	0(38)	0(29)
	66	4	14	4	17	6	2

117

Table 40 (Cont)

Food	National median	Social class (excludes unemployed and one parent families)					
		I	II	IIInm	IIIm	IV	V
Beverages:							
Fruit juices	0(480) 314	0(526) 24	68(349)	0(428) 43	0(553) 49	0(417) 18	0(387) 7
Tea	633(977)	730(889)	469(785)	500(808)	662(1,033)	1,274(1,286)	392(866)
Coffee	0(41) 328	0(26) 16	0(60) 64	0(37) 28	0(66) 68	0(17) 34	0(6) 7
Cocoa, drinking chocolate, etc	0(19) 173	0(10) 8	0(23) 51	0(18) 13	0(15) 41	0(10) 9	0(33) 5
Horlicks, Ovaltine	0(25) 191	0(18) 11	0(25) 34	0(12) 16	0(20) 31	0(35) 18	0(13) 9
Milk shakes	0(353) 18	0(0) 0	0(361) 12	0(0) 0	0(292) 1	0(0) 0	0(600) 1
Colas	0(554) 384	0(671) 12	0(832) 83	190(340)	106(217)	0(352) 23	0(487) 9
Fizzy drinks	442(653)	474(594)	450(553)	530(719)	512(663)	516(834)	290(715)
Other soft drinks	62(195)	120(313)	103(239)	90(185)	129(226)	35(130)	250(232)
Alcoholic drinks:							
Beers and lagers	0(157) 20	0(50) 4	0(224) 9	0(0) 0	0(109) 5	0(0) 0	0(0) 0
Wines	0(127) 24	0(13) 2	0(146) 7	0(197) 2	0(97) 8	0(96) 3	0(0) 0
Spirits	0(0) 0	0(0) 0	0(0) 0	0(0) 0	0(0) 0	0(0) 0	0(0) 0

118

Table 40 (Cont)

| Food | National median | Social class (excludes unemployed and one parent families) | | | | | |
		I	II	IIInm	IIIm	IV	V
Other foods:							
Pickles and sauces	10(30)	20(35)	23(36)	9(30)	10(28)	0(58)	3(34)
Soups	0(335)	0(277)	0(294)	0(303)	0(451)	30(156)	0(309)
	334	23	74	43	56	10	10
Number of children	821	51	182	93	157	70	25

Table 41: *Foods consumed by girls aged 10/11 years (g/head/week)*

Food		Region		
	Total Scotland sample	London and SE	North	Rest of GB
Number of children	424	217	262	257
Cereals:				
White bread	431(447)	354(364)	335(383)	428(450)
Brown bread	0(100)	0(96)	0(165)	0(58)
	73	22	56	33
Wholemeal bread	0(154)	0(193)	0(145)	0(21)
	90	72	65	47
Other bread	0(101)	0(127)	0(95)	0(65)
	91	49	70	73
Total bread	(518)	(466)	(479)	(497)
Bran products	0(76)	0(58)	0(79)	0(123)
	17	5	10	10
Buns and pastries	31(53)	32(61)	38(67)	19(60)
Cakes	87(115)	185(201)	91(131)	150(209)
Biscuits	144(162)	167(195)	144(157)	192(193)
Breakfast cereals	95(138)	117(146)	156(172)	153(169)
Puddings, etc	234(300)	349(397)	370(412)	294(397)
Icecream	33(61)	60(73)	46(74)	41(73)
Rice	0(134)	0(146)	0(146)	0(156)
	93	56	50	70
Pasta	48(106)	61(106)	0(217)	0(173)
			120	112

120

Table 41 (Cont)

Food	Region			
	Total Scotland sample	London and SE	North	Rest of GB
Milk and milk products:				
Cows milk, whole	1,546(1,649)	1,130(1,329)	1,327(1,496)	1,276(1,289)
Skimmed, semi skimmed milk	0(1,027)	0(910)	0(727)	0(526)
	25	5	12	7
Other milk	0(34)	0(84)	0(91)	0(324)
	91	27	58	30
Yogurt	0(243)	0(244)	0(213)	0(253)
	131	96	119	84
Cream	0(131)	0(28)	0(30)	0(21)
	108	79	108	66
Cottage cheese	0(38)	0(36)	0(32)	0(30)
	6	4	9	1
Cheese	74(111)	56(94)	38(61)	58(76)
Eggs, egg dishes	91(119)	66(94)	95(123)	90(117)
Fats and oils:				
Butter	18(36)	25(43)	8(27)	25(46)
Margarine	6(31)	0(67)	23(44)	6(31)
		103		
Low fat spread	0(31)	0(34)	0(13)	0(0)
	7	3	8	0
Vegetable oils	0(77)	0(0)	0(7)	0(10)
	7	0	6	4
Other fats and oils	0(44)	0(64)	0(24)	0(39)
	20	13	14	31

Table 41 (Cont)

Food	Total Scotland sample	Region London and SE	North	Rest of GB
Carcase meats:				
Bacon and ham	39(57)	40(56)	29(47)	36(64)
Beef and veal	114(135)	0(147) 102	43(83)	40(77)
Mutton and lamb	0(77) 16	0(113) 79	0(105) 106	0(114) 77
Pork	0(70) 27	0(96) 102	0(73) 112	0(91) 112
Other meat:				
Chicken fried in breadcrumbs	0(101) 2	0(117) 11	0(102) 1	0(77) 4
Poultry and game	38(69)	58(85)	51(75)	42(91)
Liver	0(73) 12	0(56) 46	0(65) 53	0(69) 41
Kidney	0(0) 0	0(16) 1	0(32) 6	0(190) 1
Other offals	0(73) 8	0(228) 6	0(47) 4	0(50) 9
Sausages	100(120)	68(80)	62(75)	68(89)
Burgers	0(88) 37	35(57)	0(79) 95	0(79) 111
Other meat products	199(223)	267(318)	347(360)	275(317)

Table 41 (Cont)

Food	Region			
	Total Scotland sample	London and SE	North	Rest of GB
Fish and fish products:				
Fish in batter or breadcrumbs	0(116) 30	0(123) 69	0(116) 132	0(124) 81
Fish fingers	0(88) 22	0(86) 77	0(81) 103	0(82) 125
Shellfish	0(42) 1	0(161) 6	0(39) 7	0(59) 4
Other fish	0(77) 18	0(75) 58	0(74) 116	0(81) 109
Sugar, sweets:				
Sugar	76(96)	64(91)	86(98)	103(123)
Syrup and preserves	8(26)	4(25)	12(24)	12(33)
Chocolate	100(127)	93(128)	64(92)	46(73)
Sweets	126(173)	44(98)	82(125)	66(104)
Potatoes and potato products:				
Crisps, corn snacks, etc	133(138)	109(120)	84(100)	111(114)
Chips	334(387)	294(330)	472(492)	344(379)
Potatoes	351(378)	399(417)	384(409)	423(452)

Table 41 (Cont)

Food	Region			
	Total Scotland sample	London and SE	North	Rest of GB
Vegetables:				
Carrots	0(49) 29	31(49)	44(54)	36(55)
Tomatoes	0(76) 33	0(85) 108	17(41)	10(41)
Baked beans	70(96)	100(127)	78(115)	94(122)
Peas	28(43)	40(59)	84(102)	68(87)
Salad vegetables	0(49) 34	12(34)	16(36)	10(28)
Other vegetables	68(98)	138(175)	129(140)	130(155)
Fruit:				
Citrus fruit	0(211) 35	0(275) 101	0(192) 106	0(196) 109
Apples and pears	130(207)	120(172)	132(174)	120(188)
Other fresh fruit	0(155) 34	0(153) 92	0(153) 127	0(164) 121
Other fruit	27(59)	0(136) 105	0(111) 132	0(126) 126
Nuts:				
Nuts	0(44) 8	0(44) 35	0(32) 24	0(29) 23
Peanut butter	0(38) 7	0(37) 17	0(60) 15	0(35) 27

Table 41 (Cont)

Food	Total Scotland sample	Region London and SE	North	Rest of GB
Beverages:				
Fruit juices	0(357) 27	29(276)	0(349) 74	0(581) 95
Tea	852(1,060)	642(970)	632(907)	713(1,029)
Coffee	0(55) 32	0(65) 63	0(22) 119	0(44) 114
Cocoa, drinking chocolate, etc	0(13) 10	0(25) 47	0(16) 58	0(17) 58
Horlicks, Ovaltine	0(32) 16	0(17) 31	0(26) 91	0(24) 54
Milk shakes	0(0) 0	0(396) 7	0(292) 7	0(400) 3
Colas	200(379)	128(300)	0(543) 104	0(513) 120
Fizzy drinks	359(580)	410(583)	446(676)	555(709)
Other soft drinks	76(220)	86(192)	0(395) 131	70(191)
Alcoholic drinks:				
Beers and lagers	0(0) 0	0(239) 9	0(138) 2	0(73) 8
Wines	0(122) 1	0(151) 11	0(101) 7	0(114) 5
Spirits	0(0) 0	0(0) 0	0(0) 0	0(0) 0

Table 41 (Cont)

Food	Region			
	Total Scotland sample	London and SE	North	Rest of GB
Other foods:				
Pickles and sauces	0(42) 35	10(32)	0(29)	12(30)
Soups	336(406)	0(250) 73	0(333) 127	0(270) 72
Number of children	424	217	262	257

Table 42: *Foods consumed by girls aged 10/11 years (g/head/week)*

	Family composition						
	One parent families			Two parent families			
Food	One child	Two or more children	All one parent families	One child	Two children	Three children	Four or more children
Number of children	21	88	110	120	377	141	73
Cereals:							
White bread	417(457)	376(432)	376(437)	212(324)	392(394)	434(473)	422(424)
Brown bread	0(0)	0(85)	0(86)	0(116)	0(119)	0(156)	0(61)
	0	10	10	19	69	17	8
Wholemeal bread	0(69)	0(135)	0(127)	0(197)	0(171)	0(124)	0(103)
	3	24	27	35	93	27	21
Other bread	0(109)	0(40)	0(49)	0(119)	0(59)	0(119)	0(212)
	4	22	26	46	92	25	19
Total bread	(486)	(487)	(487)	(445)	(472)	(537)	(514)
Bran products	0(0)	0(0)	0(0)	0(45)	0(97)	0(97)	0(37)
	0	0	0	2	20	5	1
Buns and pastries	24(76)	0(85)	0(92)	28(62)	33(70)	38(52)	54(63)
		40	55				
Cakes	168(162)	140(230)	145(217)	133(142)	142(172)	156(176)	140(154)
Biscuits	100(155)	155(177)	145(172)	143(154)	176(189)	160(184)	157(166)
Breakfast cereals	44(86)	156(188)	131(168)	135(142)	147(158)	113(146)	214(228)
Puddings, etc	387(459)	355(505)	361(496)	349(425)	312(352)	286(384)	279(414)
Icecream	56(96)	46(64)	46(70)	60(73)	46(75)	40(77)	31(46)
Rice	0(100)	0(98)	0(99)	0(173)	0(163)	0(139)	0(148)
	9	21	31	24	85	36	18
Pasta	0(170)	51(119)	51(112)	0(277)	0(182)	47(90)	0(150)
	10			54	173		35

127

Table 42 (Cont)

| | | Family composition | | | | | |
| | One parent families | | | Two parent families | | | |
Food	One child	Two or more children	All one parent families	One child	Two children	Three children	Four or more children
Milk and milk products:							
Cows milk, whole	903(1,667)	1,271(1,359)	1,213(1,281)	1,320(1,459)	1,332(1,416)	1,346(1,327)	1,399(1,544)
Skimmed, semi skimmed milk	0	0(1,178) / 4	0(1,165) / 4	0(136) / 3	0(749) / 19	0(0) / 0	0(929) / 2
Other milk	0(9) / 5	0(44) / 13	0(354) / 18	0(113) / 25	0(76) / 54	0(488) / 17	0(138) / 18
Yogurt	0(195) / 6	0(198) / 35	0(197) / 41	92(141)	0(231) / 141	0(211) / 46	0(297) / 28
Cream	0(23) / 8	0(18) / 32	0(19) / 40	0(19) / 48	0(35) / 123	0(21) / 38	0(24) / 23
Cottage cheese	0(0) / 0	0(36) / 3	0(36) / 3	0(41) / 4	0(28) / 8	0(0) / 0	0(0) / 0
Cheese	57(58)	44(71)	48(69)	47(82)	52(82)	40(79)	53(77)
Eggs, eggs dishes	190(163)	180(136)	114(141)	77(109)	88(110)	74(107)	95(109)
Fats and oils:							
Butter	19(48)	19(46)	19(46)	20(38)	23(39)	12(37)	16(28)
Margarine	2(27)	13(31)	10(30)	10(30)	4(33)	20(47)	35(42)
Low fat spread	0(0) / 0	0(5) / 1	0(7) / 2	0(2) / 2	0(25) / 6	0(35) / 3	0(0) / 0
Vegetable oils	0(10) / 1	0(0) / 0	0(11) / 1	0(0) / 0	0(8) / 9	0(6) / 2	0(0) / 0
Other fats and oils	0(27) / 5	0(49) / 4	0(36) / 9	0(39) / 21	0(41) / 29	0(76) / 3	0(0) / 0

Table 42 (Cont)

| | Family composition | | | | | | |
| | One parent families | | | Two parent families | | | |
Food	One child	Two or more children	All one parent families	One child	Two children	Three children	Four or more children
Carcase meats:							
Bacon and ham	30(50)	40(75)	31(70)	32(50)	38(55)	26(54)	35(51)
Beef and veal	120(97)	48(102)	54(101)	30(89)	46(87)	20(64)	24(55)
Mutton and Lamb	0(79)	0(120)	0(115)	0(136)	0(88)	0(125)	0(149)
	4	25	28	37	147	42	24
Pork	0(106)	0(116)	0(114)	0(80)	0(77)	0(92)	0(78)
	8	37	46	46	159	66	36
Other meat:							
Chicken fried in breadcrumbs	0(0)	0(0)	0(0)	0(123)	0(103)	0(97)	0(0)
	0	0	0	3	13	2	0
Poultry and Game	140(113)	20(80)	25(86)	48(76)	52(77)	41(88)	44(102)
	6	9	15	29	82	22	5
Liver	0(50)	0(57)	0(54)	0(58)	0(65)	0(79)	0(47)
Kidney	0(0)	0(23)	0(23)	0(0)	0(38)	0(0)	0(176)
	0	2	2	0	5	0	1
Other offals	0(0)	0(72)	0(75)	0(98)	0(117)	0(62)	0(54)
	0	4	4	7	11	4	2
Sausages	54(79)	58(92)	58(90)	68(79)	67(85)	66(82)	100(92)
Burgers	0(74)	0(69)	0(70)	0(87)	0(97)	28(46)	32(39)
	6	42	48	52	147		
Other meat products	232(358)	265(397)	259(309)	334(371)	317(323)	256(307)	264(288)

Table 42 (Cont)

Food	One parent families			Two parent families			
	One child	Two or more children	All one parent families	One child	Two children	Three children	Four or more children
Fish and fish products:							
Fish in batter or breadcrumbs	0(138) 7	0(149) 39	0(147) 46	0(104) 52	0(118) 143	0(117) 40	0(116) 33
Fish fingers	0(67) 5	47(51) 17	25(44) 22	0(71) 37	0(88) 51	0(84) 43	0(64) 29
Shellfish	0(0) 0	0(0) 0	0(0) 0	0(15) 5	0(52) 10	0(389) 2	0(0) 0
Other fish	0(140) 7	0(85) 17	0(101) 24	0(90) 53	0(69) 137	0(84) 62	0(51) 26
Sugar, sweets:							
Sugar	109(123)	103(129)	104(128)	52(70)	77(99)	96(118)	103(123)
Syrup and preserves	28(26)	12(34)	18(33)	4(26)	5(23)	11(33)	17(32)
Chocolate	72(102)	71(91)	71(93)	70(109)	84(107)	42(90)	9(66)
Sweets	90(148)	108(145)	106(116)	60(104)	74(111)	95(130)	58(89)
Potatoes and potato products:							
Crisps, corn snacks, etc	130(144)	112(123)	116(127)	113(126)	121(120)	92(109)	21(50)
Chips	566(551)	385(422)	392(448)	320(379)	309(382)	384(457)	344(382)
Potatoes	285(358)	411(459)	360(439)	371(415)	399(412)	412(420)	410(470)

Family composition

Table 42 (Cont)

	Family composition						
	One parent families			Two parent families			
Food	One child	Two or more children	All one parent families	One child	Two children	Three children	Four or more children
Vegetables:							
Carrots	35(57)	45(56)	44(56)	31(53)	26(45)	26(51)	66(58)
Tomatoes	0(124) / 10	35(49) / 32	33(51)	11(63)	0(66) / 183	7(41)	0(71) / 32
Baked beans	44(79)	80(103)	64(98)	106(115)	82(114)	104(126)	120(164)
Peas	63(66)	90(87)	80(83)	98(112)	56(69)	42(71)	63(102)
Salad vegetables	26(28)	10(32)	10(31)	17(48)	8(27)	5(26)	34(38)
Other vegetables	132(145)	127(162)	132(158)	158(166)	118(139)	126(148)	143(170)
Fruit:							
Citrus fruit	0(258) / 7	0(19) / 32	0(209) / 39	0(248) / 52	0(220) / 177	0(222) / 66	0(126) / 17
Apples and pears	110(114)	98(182)	98(169)	184(242)	132(180)	106(158)	58(146)
Other fresh fruit	72(82)	0(151) / 38	0(148) / 50	40(108)	0(166) / 178	0(40) / 62	0(93) / 15
Other fruit	2(67)	0(152) / 41	0(147) / 52	20(69)	0(114) / 172	12(65)	24(64)
Nuts:							
Nuts	0(26) / 7	0(31) / 13	0(29) / 20	0(25) / 20	0(46) / 31	0(47) / 15	0(271) / 4
Peanut butter	0(28) / 1	0(34) / 14	0(33) / 15	0(39) / 10	0(56) / 20	0(32) / 15	0(45) / 6

Table 42 (Cont)

Food	Family composition						
	One parent families			Two parent families			
	One child	Two or more children	All one parent families	One child	Two children	Three children	Four or more children
Beverages:							
Fruit juices	0(280) 4	0(355) 25	0(344) 29	0(558) 53	0(475) 169	0(615) 44	0(204) 20
Tea	540(1,001)	879(1,151)	662(1,120)	469(791)	600(934)	796(997)	1,110(1,244)
Coffee	8(8)	0(39) 40	0(16)	0(26) 49	0(59) 137	0(31) 56	0(21) 31
Cocoa, drinking chocolate, etc.	0(9) 3	0(16) 24	0(16) 27	0(20) 27	0(18) 73	0(29) 22	0(12) 24
Horlicks, Ovaltine	0(33) 9	0(24) 30	0(26) 39	0(15) 30	0(21) 73	0(37) 31	0(31) 17
Milk shakes	0(0) 0	0(220) 3	0(220) 3	0(400) 2	0(371) 13	0(0) 0	0(0) 0
Colas	142(309)	175(218)	165(236)	0(723) 52	0(605) 182	0(489) 64	0(375) 21
Fizzy drinks	639(803)	360(620)	424(657)	419(712)	530(692)	437(595)	290(465)
Other soft drinks	70(96) 41	0(297) 41	0(273) 53	0(344) 60	76(221)	71(235)	51(123)

Table 42 (Cont)

Food	Family composition						
	One parent families			Two parent families			
	One child	Two or more children	All one parent families	One child	Two children	Three children	Four or more children
Alcoholic drinks:							
Beers and lagers	0(0) 0	0(200) 1	0(200) 1	0(0) 0	0(218) 11	0(80) 4	0(50) 4
Wines	0(0) 0	0(30) 3	0(30) 3	0(0) 0	0(129) 17	0(177) 4	0(0) 0
Spirits	0(0) 0	0(0) 0	0(0) 0	0(0) 0	0(0) 0	0(0) 0	0(0) 0
Other foods:							
Pickles and sauces	16(21)	12(25)	13(24)	10(35)	10(29)	10(32)	4(22)
Soups	0(138) 9	0(219) 32	0(297) 42	0(328) 52	0(381) 48	0(308) 46	26(127)
Number of children	21	88	110	120	377	141	73

133

Table 43: *Foods consumed by girls aged 10/11 years (g/head/week)*

Food	Employment and benefits (benefits are also received by one parent families)				
	Father unemployed	Father in employment	Family Income Supplement (FIS)	Supplementary Benefit (SB)	Neither FIS or SB
Number of children	128	578	26	138	641
Cereals:					
White bread	467(492)	358(392)	463(473)	422(437)	362(393)
Brown bread	0(69) 9	0(126) 115	0(74) 1	0(57) 9	0(123) 114
Wholemeal bread	0(119) 16	0(165) 156	0(70) 2	0(123) 23	0(162) 175
Other bread	0(133) 39	0(82) 145	0(157) 9	0(121) 36	0(83) 164
Total bread	(552)	(474)	(535)	(494)	(478)
Bran products	0(61) 5	0(94) 24	0(0) 0	0(59) 4	0(95) 24
Buns and pastries	38(52)	37(65)	0(77) 12	19(45)	35(67)
Cakes	100(148)	148(178)	99(131)	107(157)	148(177)
Biscuits	144(171)	163(181)	128(130)	172(178)	160(181)
Breakfast cereals	127(164)	153(159)	63(132)	131(175)	146(159)
Puddings, etc	286(354)	334(402)	243(351)	380(429)	334(387)
Icecream	31(58)	52(75)	0(110)	40(62)	50(74)
Rice	0(135) 26	0(162) 136	0(135) 7	0(117) 31	0(155) 151
Pasta	72(89)	0(202) 261	0(167) 10	51(93)	0(199) 313

Table 43 (Cont)

Food	Employment and benefits (benefits are also received by one parent families)				
	Father unemployed	Father in employment	Family Income Supplement (FIS)	Supplementary Benefit (SB)	Neither FIS or SB
Milk and milk products:					
Cows milk, whole	1,106(1,153)	1,403(1,454)	890(1,034)	1,213(1,202)	1,346(1,456)
Skimmed, semi skimmed milk	0(1,025) 3	0(533) 20	0(2,217) 2	0(748) 4	0(644) 23
Other milk	0(312) 31	0(97) 83	0(29) 4	0(76) 26	0(159) 100
Yogurt	0(188) 37	0(251) 239	0(209) 9	0(172) 36	0(244) 276
Cream	0(19) 34	0(31) 197	0(31) 9	0(18) 40	0(28) 223
Cottage cheese	0(0) 0	0(33) 12	0(0) 0	0(0) 0	0(33) 15
Cheese	44(69)	52(81)	88(58)	41(71)	50(80)
Eggs, egg dishes	88(120)	80(112)	62(107)	103(117)	82(111)
Fats and oils:					
Butter	5(21)	23(41)	12(45)	8(27)	21(40)
Margarine	38(52)	4(33)	9(32)	35(46)	5(34)
Low fat spread	0(36) 2	0(2) 9	0(0) 0	0(0) 0	0(20) 12
Vegetable oils	0(11) 2	0(7) 10	0(0) 0	0(11) 1	0(8) 11
Other fats and oils	0(13) 2	0(38) 42	0(0) 0	0(69) 8	0(36) 54

Table 43 (Cont)

Food	Employment and benefits (benefits are also received by one parent families)				
	Father unemployed	Father in employment	Family Income Supplement (FIS)	Supplementary Benefit (SB)	Neither FIS or SB
Carcase meats:					
Bacon and ham	30(49)	35(58)	60(102)	30(47)	33(56)
Beef and veal	24(64)	41(85)	37(65)	28(76)	43(85)
Mutton and lamb	0(117)	0(107)	0(69)	0(120)	0(82)
	51	186	5	59	221
Pork	0(94)	0(79)	0(73)	0(105)	0(82)
	43	26	13	46	293
Other meat:					
Chicken fried in breadcrumbs	0(0)	0(105)	0(0)	0(0)	0(106)
	0	18	0	0	18
Poultry and game	42(91)	50(81)	62(107)	42(98)	46(78)
Liver	0(68)	0(64)	0(46)	0(53)	0(66)
	17	118	3	19	131
Kidney	0(0)	0(66)	0(0)	0(16)	0(67)
	0	6	0	2	7
Other offals	0(54)	0(113)	0(0)	0(58)	0(111)
	6	17	0	5	17
Sausages	64(89)	68(84)	68(97)	64(91)	68(83)
Burgers	0(76)	0(92)	0(84)	0(85)	0(88)
	54	262	12	55	293
Other meat products	320(328)	289(322)	329(336)	321(321)	275(321)

Table 43 (Cont)

Food	Employment and benefits (benefits are also received by one parent families)				
	Father unemployed	Father in employment	Family Income Supplement (FIS)	Supplementary Benefit (SB)	Neither FIS or SB
Fish and fish products:					
Fish in batter or breadcrumbs	0(102) 51	0(119) 223	0(161) 9	0(43) 133	0(119) 251
Fish fingers	0(77) 59	0(87) 208	0(50) 9	0(37)	0(87) 246
Shellfish	0(53) 2	0(86) 16	0(0) 0	0(2) 54	0(85) 16
Other fish	0(83) 42	0(73) 227	64(83)	0(95) 36	0(71) 244
Sugar, sweets:					
Sugar	104(129)	75(95)	106(122)	103(121)	76(99)
Syrup and preserves	0(43) 51	11(29)	4(14)	0(42) 64	10(29)
Chocolate	69(85)	71(104)	33(48)	69(88)	72(103)
Sweets	105(160)	60(108)	86(128)	105(151)	68(109)
Potatoes and potato products:					
Crisps, corn snacks, etc	99(109)	100(114)	57(91)	99(102)	109(116)
Chips	434(527)	309(376)	519(491)	488(505)	318(379)
Potatoes	340(397)	401(424)	524(562)	399(452)	394(410)
Vegetables:					
Carrots	30(48)	31(50)	26(33)	29(51)	31(50)
Tomatoes	20(51)	0(77) 282	42(78)	25(52)	0(75) 319
Baked beans	120(143)	80(113)	32(103)	116(143)	86(114)

137

Table 43 (Cont)

Food	Employment and benefits (benefits are also received by one parent families)				
	Father unemployed	Father in employment	Family Income Supplement (FIS)	Supplementary Benefit (SB)	Neither FIS or SB
Vegetables:					
Peas	56(86)	56(79)	55(98)	63(85)	59(78)
Salad vegetables	5(26)	16(32)	21(22)	2(22)	15(33)
Other vegetables	114(137)	132(151)	139(165)	103(150)	132(150)
Fruit:					
Citrus fruit	0(174)	0(228)	0(174)	0(195)	0(224)
	51	266	8	44	299
Apples and pears	82(136)	146(189)	19(131)	12(193)	140(163)
Other fresh fruit	0(168)	0(164)	48(57)	0(156)	0(165)
	47	266	49	49	306
Other fruit	0(118)	17(64)	30(42)	0(140)	10(54)
	45			40	
Nuts:					
Nuts	0(45)	0(38)	0(7)	0(39)	0(38)
	13	56	4	13	68
Peanut butter	0(67)	0(43)	0(30)	0(36)	0(45)
	7	47	2	7	54

138

Table 43 (Cont)

Food	Employment and benefits (benefits are also received by one parent families)				
	Father unemployed	Father in employment	Family Income Supplement (FIS)	Supplementary Benefit (SB)	Neither FIS or SB
Beverages:					
Fruit juices	0(216) 28	0(514) 256	0(470) 6	0(198) 31	0(510) 276
Tea	713(1,147)	632(944)	1,098(948)	685(1,083)	600(949)
Coffee	0(23) 55	0(48) 217	0(12) 13	0(35) 49	0(44) 262
Cocoa, drinking chocolate, etc	0(2) 25	0(19) 128	0(12) 4	0(17) 26	0(19) 143
Horlicks, Ovaltine	0(26) 37	0(24) 118	0(14) 9	0(28) 35	0(24) 144
Milk shakes	0(0) 0	0(375) 15	0(220) 3	0(0) 0	0(375) 15
Colas	0(543) 87	0(599) 259	0(415) 10	0(445) 64	0(581) 309
Fizzy drinks	318(598)	474(658)	340(613)	304(608)	459(660)
Other soft drinks	0(346) 57	90(220)	0(119) 12	0(250) 50	86(221)
Alcoholic drinks:					
Beers and lagers	0(0) 0	0(154) 19	0(0) 0	0(200) 1	0(154) 18
Wine	0(168) 3	0(121) 21	0(0) 0	0(117) 2	0(128) 22
Spirits	0(0) 0	0(0) 0	0(0) 0	0(0) 0	0(0) 0

Table 43 (Cont)

Food	Employment and benefits (benefits are also received by one parent families)				
	Father unemployed	Father in employment	Family Income Supplement (FIS)	Supplementary Benefit (SB)	Neither FIS or SB
Other foods:					
Pickles and sauces	0(44) 61	10(31)	0(33) 13	0(37) 58	13(32)
Soups	0(372) 51	0(333) 242	30(169)	0(347) 51	0(338) 265
Number of children	128	578	26	138	641

Table 44: *Food consumed by girls aged 10/11 years (g/head/week)*

Food				Type of lunch			
	Paid school meal	Free school meal	Paid school meal most days	Free school meal most days	Home	Packed lunch	Cafe
Number of children	196	137	75	32	109	263	20
Cereals:							
White bread	245(311)	391(99)	311(355)	521(505)	423(479)	437(449)	390(434)
Brown bread	0(98) 31	0(80) 15	0(79) 13	0(48) 1	0(177) 17	0(144) 43	0(32) 5
Wholemeal bread	0(97) 60	0(118) 22	0(156) 18	0(150) 3	0(153) 12	0(210) 84	0(133) 1
Other bread	0(80) 49	0(178) 26	0(103) 17	6(38)	0(71) 33	0(83) 63	0(48) 3
Total bread	(3,778)	(461)	(450)	(558)	(545)	(561)	(463)
Bran products	0(60) 6	0(0) 0	0(90) 4	0(53) 3	0(160) 6	0(76) 9	0(0) 0
Buns and pastries	38(63)	19(53)	86(91)	0(81) 15	0(103) 53	26(64)	36(81)
Cakes	192(201)	140(164)	102(111)	88(126)	106(196)	148(172)	60(120)
Biscuits	150(168)	145(168)	135(170)	171(161)	132(154)	193(211)	106(126)
Breakfast cereals	153(159)	131(169)	148(164)	84(111)	131(149)	163(171)	149(124)
Puddings, etc	362(443)	395(446)	353(431)	270(291)	372(428)	230(313)	262(396)
Icecream	55(78)	38(52)	40(62)	36(70)	41(62)	60(86)	29(60)
Rice	0(123) 62	0(95) 35	0(170) 13	0(75) 7	0(238) 29	0(173) 46	0(0) 0
Pasta	0(165) 94	100(102)	100(141)	0(215) 15	0(199) 46	0(222) 105	40(55)

Table 44 (Cont)

Food	Type of lunch						
	Paid school meal	Free school meal	Paid school meal most days	Free school meal most days	Home	Packed lunch	Cafe
Milk and milk products:							
Cows milk, whole	1,403(1,504)	907(1,082)	1,109(1,260)	1,234(1,327)	1,620(1,647)	1,365(1,470)	378(843)
Skimmed, semi skimmed milk	0(140) 9	0(1,213) 5	0(106) 1	0(0) 0	0(1,080) 2	0(1,034) 10	0(74) 1
Other milk	0(86) 34	0(302) 32	0(55) 19	0(24) 10	0(79) 9	0(134) 26	0(0) 0
Yogurt	29(105)	0(184) 39	0(146) 30	0(247) 9	0(255) 30	0(296) 113	0(41) 3
Cream	0(23) 84	0(15) 50	0(25) 32	0(37) 7	0(47) 24	0(33) 24	0(27) 1
Cottage cheese	0(0) 0	0(40) 2	0(0) 0	0(0) 0	0(0) 0	0(32) 13	0(0) 0
Cheese	48(76)	30(61)	34(78)	96(91)	50(79)	56(92)	0(114) 5
Eggs, egg dishes	90(112)	106(134)	96(131)	50(109)	97(118)	59(94)	136(167)
Fats and oils:							
Butter	18(33)	10(25)	20(27)	13(38)	39(47)	30(48)	56(60)
Margarine	5(22)	25(39)	11(38)	16(45)	0(54) 50	18(47)	0(26) 6
Low fat spread	0(18) 7	0(0) 0	0(0) 0	0(0) 0	0(36) 2	0(0) 0	0(0) 0
Vegetable oils	0(10) 5	0(0) 0	0(0) 0	0(12) 1	0(6) 5	0(0) 0	0(0) 0
Other fats and oils	0(24) 22	0(58) 14	0(47) 4	0(0) 0	0(30) 14	0(72) 9	0(0) 0

Table 44 (Cont)

Food	Type of lunch						
	Paid school meal	Free school meal	Paid school meal most days	Free school meal most days	Home	Packed lunch	Cafe
Carcase meats:							
Bacon and ham	34(52)	27(37)	45(48)	30(49)	36(80)	35(60)	104(83)
Beef and veal	54(102)	30(71)	45(92)	36(105)	45(99)	37(64)	0(167) 4
Mutton and lamb	0(102) 47	0(108) 56	0(113) 34	0(44) 32	0(119) 26	0(111) 94	0(67) 7
Pork	14(39)	0(92) 53	0(75) 31	0(95) 9	0(100) 49	0(84) 106	0(81) 5
Other meat:							
Chicken fried in breadcrumbs	0(115) 11	0(0) 0	0(103) 2	0(0) 0	0(0) 0	0(87) 5	0(0) 0
Poultry and game	52(83)	35(92)	21(74)	70(95)	34(69)	52(82)	47(87)
Liver	0(56) 40	0(72) 23	0(57) 8	0(52) 6	0(83) 15	0(60) 55	0(103) 5
Kidney	0(39) 5	0(15) 1	0(16) 1	0(0) 0	0(0) 0	0(164) 1	0(0) 0
Other offals	0(27) 4	0(53) 1	0(0) 0	0(45) 4	0(78) 7	0(154) 10	0(4) 1
Sausages	86(98)	68(46)	64(81)	52(95)	49(87)	56(66)	116(109)
Burgers	40(49)	0(80) 64	0(64) 30	0(88) 12	0(71) 30	0(97) 108	86(89)
Other meat products	289(323)	306(331)	347(423)	374(315)	297(286)	261(303)	330(351)

Table 44 (Cont)

Food	Paid school meal	Free school meal	Paid school meal most days	Free school meal most days	Home	Packed lunch	Cafe
			Type of lunch				
Fish and fish products:							
Fish in batter or breadcrumbs	0(108) 92	0(113) 45	0(124) 35	0(145) 12	0(140) 44	0(119) 83	0(141) 3
Fish fingers	30(43) 68	0(80) 68	0(100) 24	0(57) 11	0(76) 45	0(89) 73	0(77) 6
Shellfish	0(16) 4	0(0) 0	0(23) 3	0(57) 1	0(294) 3	0(46) 6	0(0) 0
Other fish	0(68) 80	0(90) 39	0(51) 26	0(120) 10	0(69) 35	0(85) 107	0(47) 6
Sugar, sweets:							
Sugar	69(82)	101(119)	53(107)	140(135)	119(135)	72(94)	65(103)
Syrup and preserves	12(24) 67	0(41) 67	3(14) 12	0(39) 12	16(42)	14(33)	0(77) 6
Chocolate	72(120)	60(88)	88(97)	85(121)	68(92)	69(89)	136(125)
Sweets	60(109)	101(157)	76(99)	112(151)	98(127)	44(92)	119(180)
Potatoes and potato products:							
Crisps, corn snacks, etc	91(99)	74(85)	62(94)	120(124)	121(132)	134(135)	122(124)
Chips	415(459)	489(550)	565(545)	323(415)	340(336)	249(267)	404(497)
Potatoes	405(441)	399(442)	426(482)	498(479)	372(388)	361(387)	550(456)

Table 44 (Cont)

Food	Type of lunch						
	Paid school meal	Free school meal	Paid school meal most days	Free school meal most days	Home	Packed lunch	Cafe
Vegetables:							
Carrots	40(48)	41(58)	31(46)	30(40)	20(42)	34(53)	16(21)
Tomatoes	6(39)	17(46)	10(44)	47(69)	0(84) 54	0(72) 118	0(87) 8
Baked beans	125(145)	127(147)	138(146)	58(90)	60(110)	40(87)	50(72)
Peas	80(90)	63(87)	74(100)	56(85)	47(65)	50(70)	50(67)
Salad vegetables	23(41)	8(27)	13(24)	4(19)	10(32)	8(32)	0(32) 7
Other vegetables	158(170)	130(157)	126(131)	73(142)	107(117)	126(151)	219(166)
Fruit:							
Citrus fruit	0(275) 75	0(181) 34	0(150) 49	0(205) 16	0(167) 45	59(133)	0(130) 6
Apples and pears	116(163)	50(132)	146(202)	132(195)	120(146)	206(234)	60(86)
Other fresh fruit	0(137) 91	0(123) 57	88(97)	0(35) 8	62(85)	0(199) 113	0(179) 3
Other fruit	18(54) 54	18(54) 54	4(60)	0(118) 15	0(150) 45	9(780)	0(123) 8
Nuts:							
Nuts	0(26) 23	0(28) 17	0(29) 5	0(38) 5	0(41) 10	0(48) 28	0(0) 0
Peanut butter	0(42) 13	0(53) 10	0(0) 0	0(46) 2	0(48) 11	0(35) 30	0(0) 0

145

Table 44 (Cont)

Food	Type of lunch						
	Paid school meal	Free school meal	Paid school meal most days	Free school meal most days	Home	Packed lunch	Cafe
Beverages:							
Fruit juices	0(417) 74	0(261) 31	0(626) 29	0(106) 5	0(551) 36	8(279)	0(340) 2
Tea	662(983)	540(854)	416(830)	1,185(1,362)	1,296(1,499)	392(803)	547(731)
Coffee	0(45) 87	0(14) 59	0(20) 26	2(20)	0(37) 45	0(63) 92	0(53) 2
Cocoa, drinking chocolate, etc	0(11) 55	0(20) 36	0(13) 13	0(0) 0	0(8) 11	0(28) 56	0(0) 0
Horlicks, Ovaltine	0(23) 70	0(29) 43	0(18) 22	0(21) 15	0(31) 22	0(30) 14	0(8) 5
Milk shakes	0(374) 8	0(220) 3	0(0) 0	0(0) 0	0(292) 1	0(400) 5	0(0) 0
Colas	0(688) 83	0(455) 60	0(806) 36	150(207)	0(382) 47	0(536) 124	334(459)
Fizzy drinks	498(670)	364(553)	530(827)	212(416)	406(779)	450(637)	530(637)
Other soft drinks	36(103)	0(269) 59	62(175)	0(210) 15	0(425) 49	266(318)	200(296)
Alcoholic drinks:							
Beers and lagers	0(123) 9	0(0) 0	0(0) 0	0(192) 2	0(0) 0	0(187) 8	0(0) 0
Wines	0(91) 5	0(168) 3	0(10) 1	0(0) 0	0(184) 2	0(121) 8	0(0) 0
Spirits	0(0) 0	0(0) 0	0(0) 0	0(0) 0	0(0) 0	0(0) 0	0(0) 0

Table 44 (Cont)

Food	Type of lunch						
	Paid school meal	Free school meal	Paid school meal most days	Free school meal most days	Home	Packed lunch	Cafe
Other foods:							
Pickles and sauces	19(36)	4(22)	0(30) 28	0(40) 13	3(21)	9(30)	100(60)
Soups	0(224) 72	0(279) 43	170(182)	0(458) 16	170(266)	0(345) 87	0(682) 5
Number of children	196	137	75	32	109	263	20

147

Table 45: *Foods consumed by girls aged 10/11 years (g/head/week)*

Food	Type of school meal (excluding those not taking a school meal)		
	Cafeteria	Fixed price	Other
Number of children	25	388	23
Cereals:			
White bread	225(213)	360(375)	120(266)
Brown bread	0(0)	0(91)	0(45)
	0	56	4
Wholemeal bread	0(163)	0(108)	0(96)
	12	82	10
Other bread	0(0)	0(107)	0(68)
	0	105	4
Total bread	(295)	(440)	(387)
Bran products	0(95)	0(52)	0(0)
	5	8	0
Buns and Pastries	70(127)	38(60)	0(125)
			6
Cakes	133(161)	142(168)	140(186)
Biscuits	167(207)	143(168)	133(128)
Breakfast cereals	54(117)	140(164)	153(119)
Puddings, etc	225(370)	370(441)	254(317)
Icecream	60(51)	44(69)	52(44)
Rice	0(102)	0(117)	54(66)
	10	96	
Pasta	0(252)	66(100)	0(151)
	11		9
Milk and milk products:			
Cows milk, whole	1,346(1,163)	1,129(1,320)	1,530(1,419)
Skimmed, semi skimmed milk	0(0)	0(493)	0(0)
	0	15	0
Other milk	0(144)	0(153)	0(11)
	8	83	5
Yogurt	0(222)	0(188)	0(244)
	11	155	10
Cream	0(35)	0(21)	0(27)
	4	162	8
Cottage cheese	0(0)	0(42)	0(0)
	0	2	0
Cheese	25(68)	43(73)	59(80)
Eggs, egg dishes	104(126)	92(119)	134(171)
Fats and oils:			
Butter	19(21)	16(31)	16(26)
Margarine	45(41)	11(32)	8(28)
Low fat spread	0(0)	0(16)	0(0)
	0	8	0
Vegetable oils	0(0)	0(10)	0(10)
	0	3	4
Other fats and oils	0(0)	0(38)	0(0)
	0	38	0

Table 45 (Cont)

Food	Type of school meal (excluding those not taking a school meal)		
	Cafeteria	Fixed price	Other
Carcase meats:			
Bacon and ham	45(58)	31(46)	32(47)
Beef and veal	21(46)	44(95)	40(69)
Mutton and lamb	0(134)	0(103)	0(96)
	8	136	11
Pork	0(97)	0(81)	0(89)
	11	169	10
Other meat:			
Chicken fried in breadcrumbs	0(0)	0(113)	0(0)
	0	12	0
Poultry and game	34(76)	43(84)	98(117)
Liver	0(44)	0(62)	0(73)
	8	68	2
Kidney	0(0)	0(31)	0(0)
	0	7	0
Other offals	0(0)	0(44)	0(0)
	0	9	0
Sausages	74(91)	78(94)	83(102)
Burgers	34(46)	0(85)	40(41)
		182	
Other meat products	440(483)	321(335)	265(318)
Fish and fish products:			
Fish in batter or breadcrumbs	0(234)	0(113)	0(105)
	4	168	11
Fish fingers	0(105)	0(83)	25(34)
	8	181	
Shellfish	0(0)	0(28)	0(0)
	0	8	0
Other fish	0(32)	0(77)	0(57)
	5	140	9
Sugar, sweets:			
Sugar	65(108)	81(101)	72(110)
Syrup and preserves	0(45)	4(20)	12(22)
	9		
Chocolate	41(94)	75(109)	72(74)
Sweets	20(55)	81(130)	71(129)
Potatoes and potato products:			
Crisps, corn snacks, etc	84(79)	84(98)	53(76)
Chips	460(575)	448(504)	295(319)
Potatoes	453(539)	400(443)	515(492)
Vegetables:			
Carrots	14(30)	35(51)	33(59)
Tomatoes	30(38)	13(45)	0(78)
			11
Baked beans	176(189)	120(139)	86(141)
Peas	58(54)	74(95)	50(53)
Salad vegetables	14(24)	12(32)	17(36)
Other vegetables	175(162)	132(156)	218(176)

149

Table 45 (Cont)

Food	Type of school meal (excluding those not taking a school meal)		
	Cafeteria	Fixed price	Other
Fruit:			
Citrus fruit	0(134)	0(238)	0(144)
	9	132	9
Apples and pears	146(192)	104(156)	134(230)
Other fresh fruit	18(70)	0(143)	0(82)
		179	7
Other fruit	44(65)	0(106)	0(119)
		194	10
Nuts:			
Nuts	0(0)	0(27)	0(38)
	0	46	5
Peanut butter	0(0)	0(50)	0(8)
	0	23	2
Beverages:			
Fruit juices	100(271)	0(396)	0(532)
		116	10
Tea	559(682)	540(919)	1,484(1,636)
Coffee	0(22)	0(30)	0(72)
	7	173	8
Cocoa, drinking chocolate, etc	0(27)	0(14)	0(13)
	6	91	8
Horlicks, Ovaltine	0(13)	0(24)	0(27)
	3	143	5
Milk shakes	0(0)	0(337)	0(0)
	0	11	0
Colas	115(506)	0(605)	200(244)
		171	
Fizzy drinks	660(840)	416(637)	360(514)
Other soft drinks	35(128)	0(244)	51(96)
		191	
Alcoholic drinks:			
Beers and lagers	0(0)	0(187)	0(50)
	0	7	4
Wines	0(144)	0(87)	0(0)
	3	6	0
Spirits	0(0)	0(0)	0(0)
	0	0	0
Other foods:			
Pickles and sauces	20(26)	10(38)	20(46)
Soups	0(277)	0(279)	0(358)
	7	160	7
Number of children	25	388	23

Table 46: *Foods consumed by boys aged 14/15 years (g/head/week)*

Food	National median	Social class (excludes unemployed and one parent families)					
		I	II	III nm	III m	IV	V
Number of children	513	33	103	32	125	59	11
Cereals:							
White bread	610(670)	522(509)	517(545)	689(824)	621(691)	746(734)	783(745)
Brown bread	0(209)	0(284)	0(288)	0(296)	0(176)	0(120)	0(124)
	94	13	26	3	18	12	2
Wholemeal bread	0(234)	0(345)	0(248)	0(275)	0(250)	0(138)	0(513)
	106	10	36	3	22	10	1
Other bread	0(210)	0(86)	0(122)	0(268)	0(183)	0(76)	0(0)
	120	13	20	13	28	15	0
Total bread	(806)	(754)	(729)	(989)	(802)	(801)	840
Bran products	0(209)	0(170)	0(345)	0(377)	0(231)	0(66)	0(0)
	20	3	3	3	3	2	0
Buns and pastries	0(135)	0(122)	0(143)	0(170)	0(130)	48(71)	40(88)
	249	15	51	11	57		
Cakes	130(189)	174(235)	173(223)	170(248)	114(192)	161(186)	104(114)
Biscuits	153(195)	186(243)	165(209)	119(199)	155(196)	201(225)	64(102)
Breakfast cereals	220(254)	343(387)	244(242)	202(224)	218(250)	167(266)	107(141)
Puddings, etc	287(265)	388(427)	299(371)	370(484)	312(399)	290(340)	128(241)
Icecream	0(129)	0(166)	0(143)	0(133)	0(123)	0(104)	0(88)
	173	10	36	13	46	24	4
Rice	0(279)	0(296)	0(188)	0(225)	0(254)	0(292)	0(99)
	121	6	36	12	23	15	2
Pasta	0(275)	0(288)	0(272)	0(270)	0(306)	0(214)	0(141)
	182	16	45	12	44	16	2

Table 46 (Cont)

Food	National median	Social class (excludes unemployed and one parent families)					
		I	II	III nm	III m	IV	V
Milk and milk products:							
Cows milk, whole	1,710(1,905)	2,814(2,527)	1,830(2,033)	1,660(2,151)	1,803(1,990)	1,609(1,752)	1,242(1,526)
Skimmed, semi skimmed milk	0(1,099) 11	0(0) 0	0(0) 0	0(358) 3	0(1,256) 2	0(0) 0	0(0) 0
Other milk	0(125) 67	0(61) 3	0(59) 12	0(188) 2	0(293) 11	0(105) 11	0(32) 2
Yogurt	0(254) 118	0(269) 7	0(258) 42	0(265) 8	0(238) 23	0(247) 14	0(0) 2
Cream	0(35) 114	0(47) 9	0(31) 27	0(26) 11	0(42) 25	0(50) 12	0(0) 0
Cottage cheese	0(0) 0	0(0) 0	0(0) 0	0(0) 0	0(0) 0	0(0) 0	0(0) 0
Cheese	82(137)	122(168)	138(171)	94(136)	69(117)	46(90)	0(114) 5
Eggs, egg dishes	114(158)	126(177)	103(160)	80(168)	110(152)	115(131)	196(221)
Fats and oils:							
Butter	33(63)	22(54)	46(69)	36(71)	41(69)	65(84)	0(84) 5
Margarine	6(41)	10(64)	5(34)	24(64)	4(36)	0(56) 22	0(118) 5
Low fat spread	0(28) 6	0(0) 0	0(36) 4	0(18) 1	0(0) 0	0(0) 0	0(0) 0
Vegetable oils	0(19) 17	0(42) 2	0(21) 8	0(25) 1	0(6) 3	0(0) 0	0(0) 0
Other fats and oils	0(73) 22	0(61) 5	0(120) 5	0(25) 3	0(100) 2	0(31) 2	0(0) 0

Table 46 (Cont)

Food	National median	Social class (excludes unemployed and one parent families)					
		I	II	III nm	III m	IV	V
Carcase meats:							
Bacon and ham	44(73)	25(64)	63(81)	37(105)	56(86)	25(53)	64(62)
Beef and veal	48(111)	0(260) 16	90(127)	0(120) 16	62(127)	56(94)	0(260) 5
Mutton and lamb	0(180) 173	47(45) 11	0(125) 32	0(446) 11	0(155) 36	0(118) 24	0(84) 4
Pork	0(126) 211	58(83)	0(132) 44	0(145) 14	0(126) 61	0(116) 25	0(117) 5
Other meat:							
Chicken fried in breadcrumbs	0(127) 9	0(0) 0	0(144) 2	0(140) 2	0(0) 0	0(0) 0	0(0) 0
Poultry and game	90(117)	67(131)	115(149)	94(114)	90(115)	112(118)	116(111)
Liver	0(112) 109	0(90) 11	0(128) 21	0(208) 5	0(92) 28	0(103) 15	0(152) 2
Kidney	0(67) 9	0(0) 0	0(97) 2	0(16) 2	0(16) 1	0(83) 2	0(0) 0
Other offals	0(59) 14	0(2) 2	0(0) 0	0(84) 2	0(49) 4	0(78) 3	0(0) 0
Sausages	102(133)	58(108)	90(132)	190(176)	113(139)	104(152)	182(225)
Burgers	36(72)	46(72)	0(133) 43	45(108)	40(74)	42(78)	0(99) 3
Other meat products	401(468)	305(459)	399(450)	364(430)	458(500)	400(469)	367(383)

153

Table 46 (Cont)

Food	National median	Social class (excludes unemployed and one parent families)					
		I	II	III nm	III m	IV	V
Fish and fish products:							
Fish in batter or breadcrumbs	0(156) 160	0(130) 5	0(138) 32	0(195) 5	0(156) 37	0(134) 18	0(189) 8
Fish fingers	0(113) 129	0(83) 7	0(130) 24	0(0) 0	0(110) 37	0(82) 19	0(209) 3
Shellfish	0(67) 21	0(0) 0	0(93) 7	0(113) 1	0(69) 3	0(39) 4	0(0) 0
Other fish	0(109) 171	0(113) 12	0(107) 44	0(130) 9	0(105) 34	0(91) 17	0(90) 5
Sugar, sweets:							
Sugar	175(205)	183(207)	155(163)	178(206)	175(216)	203(226)	175(197)
Syrup and preserves	0(72) 235	34(45)	10(36)	4(41)	0(84) 61	0(55) 20	0(67) 4
Chocolate	106(169)	114(193)	108(158)	251(317)	96(148)	83(174)	84(88)
Sweets	16(68)	37(83)	0(140) 46	4(57)	30(86)	19(82)	12(72)
Potatoes and potato products:							
Crisps, corn snacks, etc	55(80)	63(77)	56(75)	53(78)	67(86)	56(89)	77(88)
Chips	690(762)	320(486)	564(663)	620(714)	597(694)	618(786)	766(913)
Potatoes	540(589)	556(587)	480(543)	580(655)	616(631)	584(594)	674(765)

154

Table 46 (Cont)

Food	Social class (excludes unemployed and one parent families)						
	National median	I	II	III nm	III m	IV	V
Vegetables:							
Carrots	20(54)	51(73)	32(61)	56(66)	7(50)	15(46)	56(79)
Tomatoes	0(103)	60(65)	0(109)	24(48)	0(94)	0(124)	21(88)
	189		38		46	15	
Baked beans	146(233)	106(141)	150(228)	96(181)	130(223)	176(254)	50(265)
Peas	85(110)	65(92)	66(86)	68(100)	84(111)	108(130)	84(105)
Salad vegetables	0(58)	0(72)	0(63)	21(38)	0(56)	0(47)	0(86)
	182	15	40		42	13	4
Other vegetables	146(200)	288(316)	181(219)	210(246)	167(216)	124(148)	180(192)
Fruit:							
Citrus fruit	0(235)	62(111)	0(327)	0(303)	0(210)	0(267)	0(171)
	179		41	42	42	17	3
Apples and pears	0(306)	0(267)	30(165)	0(427)	81(146)	0(321)	127(177)
	241	14		17		25	
Other fresh fruit	0(155)	64(84)	0(148)	0(118)	0(152)	0(214)	0(174)
	148		45	9	29	10	3
Other fruit	0(163)	0(168)	0(201)	0(150)	0(148)	0(133)	0(111)
	178	13	49	13	41	20	2
Nuts:							
Nuts	0(60)	0(45)	0(49)	0(0)	0(80)	0(47)	0(0)
	44	7	8	0	15	5	0
Peanut butter	0(49)	0(50)	0(40)	0(45)	0(43)	0(35)	0(58)
	37	7	8	2	4	3	1

155

Table 46 (Cont)

Food	National median	Social class (excludes unemployed and one parent families)					
		I	II	III nm	III m	IV	V
Beverages:							
Fruit juices	0(415)	0(781)	0(448)	0(373)	0(326)	0(275)	0(384)
	132	10	37	8	34	11	2
Tea	1,487(1,748)	1,517(1,869)	1,024(1,442)	1,851(1,991)	1,452(1,711)	953(1,802)	2,275(2,099)
Coffee	4(58)	6(260)	2(48)	4(23)	7(74)	0(61)	6(12)
						29	
Cocoa, drinking chocolate, etc.	0(26)	0(28)	0(34)	0(13)	0(24)	0(33)	0(41)
	79	6	10	8	23	6	3
Horlicks, Ovaltine	0(36)	0(13)	0(23)	0(16)	0(46)	0(21)	0(52)
	86	3	9	5	19	12	1
Milk shakes	0(322)	0(330)	0(0)	0(0)	0(330)	0(0)	0(0)
	3	1	0	0	1	0	0
Colas	0(704)	200(394)	0(742)	185(374)	0(617)	0(734)	0(609)
	208		42		53	21	3
Fizzy drinks	250(522)	138(392)	310(454)	434(689)	200(576)	250(600)	182(328)
Other soft drinks	0(319)	44(253)	0(292)	41(129)	0(254)	0(314)	0(252)
	219		50		46	26	4
Alcoholic drinks:							
Beers and lagers	0(785)	0(830)	0(719)	0(471)	0(841)	0(612)	0(168)
	51	7	12	5	9	5	2
Wines	0(180)	0(305)	0(71)	0(149)	0(125)	0(0)	0(0)
	35	6	15	3	5	0	0
Spirits	0(53)	0(0)	0(60)	0(0)	0(0)	0(33)	0(0)
	8	0	1	0	0	2	0

Table 46 (Cont)

Food	National median	Social class (excludes unemployed and one parent families)					
		I	II	III nm	III m	IV	V
Other foods:							
Pickles and sauces	10(46)	50(72)	12(54)	15(48)	5(32)	8(48)	0(102) 5
Soups	0(458) 244	230(362)	168(252)	0(457) 12	0(417) 60	26(232)	0(227) 5
Number of children	513	33	103	32	125	59	11

157

Table 47: *Foods consumed by boys aged 14/15 years (g/head/week)*

Food	Region			
	Total Scotland sample	London and SE	North	Rest of GB
Number of children	56	145	149	162
Cereals:				
White bread	559(621)	645(669)	605(653)	621(695)
Brown bread	0(189) 6	0(271) 29	0(188) 33	0(173) 26
Wholemeal bread	0(199) 13	0(245) 32	0(225) 29	0(246) 32
Other bread	0(320) 7	0(227) 40	0(224) 42	0(146) 31
Total bread	(723)	(839)	(812)	(799)
Bran products	0(0) 0	0(341) 4	0(150) 5	0(185) 11
Buns and pastries	0(109) 19	0(160) 72	22(69)	0(21) 81
Cakes	110(154)	136(202)	103(170)	164(207)
Biscuits	107(164)	169(195)	148(190)	163(211)
Breakfast cereals	202(218)	197(243)	230(271)	238(259)
Puddings, etc	202(311)	244(356)	307(388)	310(370)
Icecream	0(152) 27	0(132) 52	0(117) 39	0(122) 55
Rice	0(182) 11	0(250) 48	0(374) 28	0(275) 35
Pasta	0(248) 20	0(273) 58	0(251) 51	0(310) 53

Table 47 (Cont)

Food	Total Scotland sample	Region		
		London and SE	North	Rest of GB
Milk and milk products:				
Cows milk, whole	2,033(2,171)	1,445(1,773)	1,719(1,837)	1,803(1,992)
Skimmed, semi skimmed milk	0(1,144)	0(619)	0(1,931)	0(820)
	1	1	1	6
Other milk	0(40)	0(153)	0(120)	0(12)
	41	18	29	15
Yogurt	0(260)	0(245)	0(269)	0(254)
	8	40	24	45
Cream	0(36)	0(33)	0(37)	0(36)
	14	34	27	39
Cottage cheese	0(0)	0(0)	0(0)	0(0)
	0	0	0	0
Cheese	122(168)	90(148)	82(135)	72(118)
Eggs, egg dishes	105(162)	100(147)	120(170)	124(155)
Fats and oils:				
Butter	27(38)	50(76)	21(55)	43(68)
Margarine	9(47)	0(90)	8(42)	7(37)
		65		
Low fat spread	0(0)	0(6)	0(0)	0(39)
	0	2	0	4
Vegetable oils	0(0)	0(27)	0(6)	0(17)
	0	6	3	8
Other fats and oils	0(7)	0(73)	0(96)	0(76)
	6	5	1	10

Table 47 (Cont)

Food	Region			
	Total Scotland sample	London and SE	North	Rest of GB
Carcase meat:				
Bacon and ham	31(50)	42(70)	44(69)	46(86)
Beef and veal	166(190)	0(174) 71	68(114)	0(213) 79
Mutton and lamb	0(145) 13	0(213) 60	0(196) 53	0(188) 47
Pork	0(94) 23	0(134) 55	0(139) 57	0(137) 76
Other meats:				
Chicken fried in breadcrumbs	0(134) 4	0(113) 3	0(36) 1	0(0) 0
Poultry and game	68(100)	96(128)	80(108)	94(122)
Liver	0(156) 11	0(87) 40	0(119) 24	0(121) 71
Kidney	0(0) 0	0(87) 3	0(16) 2	0(76) 4
Other offals	0(78) 6	0(47) 3	0(46) 2	0(41) 3
Sausages	186(196)	112(141)	86(110)	91(127)
Burgers	0(114) 24	70(10)	46(74)	0(123) 71
Other meat products	305(365)	368(424)	450(513)	446(502)

Table 47 (Cont)

Food	Total Scotland sample	Region		
		London and SE	North	Rest of GB
Fish and fish products:				
Fish in batter or breadcrumbs	64(84)	0(169) 31	0(153) 61	0(146) 39
Fish fingers	0(125) 6	0(111) 30	0(103) 39	0(119) 54
Shellfish	0(145) 4	0(42) 7	0(46) 6	0(68) 4
Other fish	0(106) 14	0(119) 44	0(115) 54	0(48) 60
Sugar, sweets:				
Sugar	180(201)	162(192)	158(192)	204(230)
Syrup and preserves	0(77) 23	0(60) 62	0(72) 69	0(78) 81
Chocolate	187(249)	77(163)	92(158)	106(157)
Sweets	0(87) 14	0(124) 44	0(67) 54	0(68) 60
Potatoes and potato products:				
Crisps, corn snacks, etc	77(100)	54(76)	28(66)	72(91)
Chips	832(849)	468(558)	954(990)	632(706)
Potatoes	478(524)	644(632)	386(478)	576(676)

161

Table 47 (Cont)

Food	Total Scotland sample	Region		
		London and SE	North	Rest of GB
Vegetables:				
Carrots	0(54) 21	24(56)	50(65)	29(54)
Tomatoes	0(55) 19	0(104) 47	0(107) 47	0(113) 76
Baked beans	130(267)	166(229)	134(209)	148(246)
Peas	55(75)	77(105)	88(120)	104(118)
Salad vegetables	0(36) 15	0(76) 57	0(48) 39	0(54) 71
Other vegetables	80(120)	197(255)	121(175)	153(203)
Fruit:				
Citrus fruit	0(208) 15	0(261) 51	0(209) 46	0(239) 67
Apples and pears	0(219) 23	0(320) 71	0(123) 67	0(344) 80
Other fresh fruit	0(136) 22	0(178) 36	0(136) 32	0(158) 58
Other fruit	0(111) 17	0(138) 53	0(163) 48	0(202) 60
Nuts:				
Nuts	0(32) 2	0(83) 13	0(45) 15	0(59) 13
Peanut butter	0(21) 2	0(50) 13	0(41) 5	0(54) 17

Table 47 (Cont)

Food	Total Scotland sample	Region		
		London and SE	North	Rest of GB
Beverages:				
Fruit juices	0(466) 13	0(576) 43	0(319) 27	0(314) 48
Tea	1,318(1,576)	1,502(1,738)	1,720(1,783)	1,342(1,783)
Coffee	6(20)	3(102)	4(36)	3(51)
Cocoa, drinking chocolate, etc	0(38) 5	0(25) 26	0(34) 21	0(26) 27
Horlicks, Ovaltine	0(41) 11	0(24) 25	0(48) 27	0(53) 23
Milk shakes	0(0) 0	0(316) 2	0(0) 0	0(330) 1
Colas	0(826) 21	0(721) 70	0(656) 58	0(690) 60
Fizzy drinks	200(663)	328(569)	330(521)	150(435)
Other soft drinks	0(786) 25	35(128)	0(325) 48	0(230) 70
Alcoholic drinks:				
Beers and lagers	0(743) 4	0(116) 14	0(570) 13	0(698) 20
Wines	0(184) 1	0(206) 15	0(181) 10	0(129) 8
Spirits	0(0) 0	0(0) 0	0(28) 4	0(83) 3

163

Table 47 (Cont)

Food	Total Scotland sample	Region		
		London and SE	North	Rest of GB
Other foods:				
Pickles and sauces	0(26) 22	16(56)	10(44)	9(44)
Soups	400(504)	0(405) 63	0(471) 58	0(401) 76
Number of children	56	145	149	162

164

Table 48: *Foods consumed by boys aged 14/15 years (g/head/week)*

Food	Family composition						
	One parent families		All one parent families	Two parent families			
	One child	Two or more children		One child	Two children	Three children	Four or more children
Number of children	49	31	80	207	131	58	37
Cereals:							
White bread	662(752)	526(606)	556(695)	559(646)	660(661)	698(776)	591(614)
Brown bread	0(169)	0(124)	0(140)	0(222)	0(260)	0(84)	0(263)
	7	6	13	38	29	11	4
Wholemeal bread	0(80)	0(210)	0(134)	0(289)	0(202)	0(225)	0(207)
	8	5	13	46	28	12	7
Other bread	0(181)	0(330)	0(268)	0(143)	0(96)	0(140)	0(694)
	5	8	13	47	34	11	15
Total bread	(809)	(746)	(785)	(784)	(787)	(863)	(951)
Bran products	0(190)	0(0)	0(190)	0(152)	0(336)	0(74)	0(0)
	4	0	4	7	7	2	0
Buns and pastries	28(82)	0(161)	0(163)	0(135)	21(61)	24(69)	40(72)
		15	39	94			
Cakes	112(189)	119(133)	112(167)	110(176)	174(216)	159(200)	72(196)
Biscuits	182(215)	90(121)	132(178)	143(189)	192(228)	134(194)	140(151)
Breakfast cereals	212(225)	230(281)	213(247)	203(227)	238(286)	307(327)	130(185)
Puddings, etc	284(370)	218(323)	234(352)	246(232)	432(459)	287(421)	87(203)
Icecream	0(156)	0(87)	0(130)	0(137)	0(117)	0(100)	0(189)
	15	9	24	63	51	24	11
Rice	0(225)	0(308)	0(254)	0(232)	0(352)	0(222)	0(465)
	10	5	15	57	35	9	6
Pasta	0(236)	0(243)	0(241)	0(270)	0(247)	0(283)	0(259)
	13	7	21	75	51	20	16

Table 48 (Cont)

	Family composition						
	One parent families			Two parent families			
Food	One child	Two or more children	All one parent families	One child	Two children	Three children	Four or more children
Milk and milk products:							
Cows milk, whole	1,593(1,923)	1,092(1,277)	1,408(1,770)	1,630(1,893)	2,033(2,110)	1765(2,021)	1,800(1,868)
Skimmed, semi skimmed milk	0(0) 0	0(2,443) 1	0(1,562) 2	0(1,289) 3	0(913) 5	0(0) 0	0(0) 0
Other milk	0(97) 12	0(142) 3	0(108) 15	0(124) 20	0(111) 22	0(329) 5	0(23) 4
Yogurt	0(228) 13	0(492) 1	0(254) 14	0(212) 48	0(328) 33	0(262) 14	0(178) 7
Cream	0(42) 9	0(31) 7	0(37) 16	0(38) 43	0(30) 32	0(45) 16	0(20) 7
Cottage cheese	0(0) 0	0(0) 0	0(0) 0	0(0) 0	0(0) 0	0(0) 0	0(0) 0
Cheese	68(113)	86(187)	75(142)	79(130)	112(144)	63(118)	101(169)
Eggs, egg dishes	126(156)	76(133)	107(147)	101(165)	117(149)	157(164)	102(164)
Fats and oils:							
Butter	23(35)	16(47)	23(40)	42(71)	50(71)	46(67)	24(38)
Margarine	10(57)	20(47)	15(53)	0(68) 100	7(41)	0(90) 25	24(57)
Low fat spread	0(0) 0	0(0) 0	0(0) 0	0(28) 6	0(0) 0	0(0) 0	0(0) 0
Vegetable oils	0(0) 0	0(0) 0	0(21) 2	0(16) 9	0(42) 2	0(10) 2	0(15) 3
Other fats and oils	0(105) 2	0(0) 0	0(105) 2	0(49) 6	0(80) 14	0(61) 3	0(0) 0

Table 48 (Cont)

Food	One parent families			Two parent families			
	One child	Two or more children	All one parent families	One child	Two children	Three children	Four or more children
Carcase meats:							
Bacon and ham	40(73)	45(52)	40(65)	60(79)	46(73)	30(81) 18	0(75)
Beef and veal	46(117)	0(200) 9	0(222) 34	74(115)	41(120)	63(119)	0(202) 14
Mutton and lamb	0(131) 17	0(208) 6	0(151) 23	0(165) 79	0(134) 37	0(122) 17	0(445) 17
Pork	0(110) 19	0(103) 11	0(108) 30	0(140) 91	0(118) 37	0(102) 21	0(147) 12
Other meat:							
Chicken fried in breadcrumbs	0(118) 2	0(36) 1	0(86) 3	0(139) 4	0(0) 0	0(175) 2	0(0) 0
Poultry and game	86(95) 9	81(128) 6	81(108) 16	86(123) 49	90(110) 25	112(122) 12	90(122) 7
Liver	0(105) 6	0(138)	0(119)	0(124)	0(106)	0(73)	0(100)
Kidney	0(110) 1	0(0) 0	0(110) 1	0(116) 3	0(91) 4	0(0) 0	0(0) 0
Other offals	0(0) 0	0(50) 2	0(50) 2	0(60) 8	0(42) 4	0(67) 3	0(0) 0
Sausages	114(120)	112(123)	112(121) 17	104(133) 104	114(143) 65	102(139)	80(120) 0
Burgers	60(84)	70(73)	60(80)	0(140)	0(143)	42(74)	0(138)
Other meat products	463(514)	404(470)	450(497)	308(451)	400(470)	462(539)	296(390)

Family composition

167

Table 48 (Cont)

Food	One parent families			Two parent families			
	One child	Two or more children	All one parent families	One child	Two children	Three children	Four or more children
Fish and fish products:							
Fish in batter or breadcrumbs	0(219) 15	0(173) 14	0(196) 29	0(141) 62	0(157) 41	0(129) 19	0(128) 10
Fish fingers	0(108) 13	0(170) 9	0(133) 20	0(112) 43	0(93) 30	0(120) 22	0(116) 10
Shellfish	0(34) 2	0(0) 0	0(44) 3	0(75) 13	0(25) 2	0(142) 1	0(60) 2
Other fish	0(92) 18	0(92) 10	0(92) 28	0(113) 71	0(120) 45	0(97) 19	0(112) 7
Sugar, sweets:							
Sugar	152(188)	135(199)	146(193)	176(203)	169(202)	197(229)	194(219)
Syrup and preserves	0(101) 19	0(40) 14	0(76) 33	0(82) 90	10(36)	0(50) 25	0(61) 16
Chocolate	144(188)	68(125)	105(164)	106(150)	47(173)	119(186)	167(247)
Sweets	24(59)	26(42)	25(53)	8(65)	19(80)	8(70)	16(66)
Potatoes and potato products:							
Crisps, corn snacks, etc	53(96)	24(45)	48(76)	53(83)	75(80)	59(87)	50(62)
Chips	822(909)	822(940)	834(921)	583(690)	624(713)	690(775)	826(971)
Potatoes	388(520)	509(561)	414(536)	568(637)	566(589)	549(580)	360(451)

Family composition

Table 48 (Cont)

	Family composition						
	One parent families			Two parent families			
Food	One child	Two or more children	All one parent families	One child	Two children	Three children	Four or more children
Vegetables:							
Carrots	20(48)	45(62)	39(54)	20(58)	88(57)	13(49)	0(66) 16
Tomatoes	0(100) 18	0(109) 13	0(163) 31	0(104) 75	98(48)	0(100) 18	0(69) 7
Baked beans	224(321)	192(226)	200(284)	138(234)	108(183)	214(246)	214(270)
Peas	100(110)	82(127)	90(115)	92(108)	72(103)	60(110)	76(139)
Salad vegetables	0(61) 18	0(57) 9	0(58) 27	0(53) 76	0(55) 55	0(92) 14	0(68) 9
Other vegetables	136(176)	118(161)	120(170)	162(199)	181(223)	121(184)	133(220)
Fruit:							
Citrus fruit	0(234) 16	0(123) 9	0(195) 25	0(262) 73	0(231) 51	0(211) 21	0(204) 1
Apples and pears	0(301) 21	0(146) 11	0(264) 32	0(317) 103	69(171)	0(241) 28	0(339) 11
Other fresh fruit	0(137) 11	0(112) 6	0(128) 16	0(172) 65	0(144) 50	0(176) 10	0(94) 6
Other fruit	0(220) 13	0(70) 8	0(161) 21	0(141) 74	0(208) 50	0(137) 21	0(158) 12

169

Table 48 (Cont)

Food	Family composition						
	One parent families			Two parent families			
	One child	Two or more children	All one parent families	One child	Two children	Three children	Four or more children
Nuts:							
Nuts	0(98) 4	0(0) 0	0(85) 5	0(64) 15	0(47) 13	0(49) 9	0(107) 2
Peanut butter	0(48) 4	0(70) 2	0(54) 6	0(56) 12	0(38) 12	0(0) 0	0(12) 1
Beverages:							
Fruit juices	0(412) 16	0(417) 5	0(413) 21	0(380) 51	0(460) 43	0(519) 12	0(122) 5
Tea	576(1,478)	1,302(1,526)	777(1,496)	1,773(1,873)	1,389(1,698)	1,710(1,892)	1,849(2,096)
Coffee	2(41)	3(36)	3(39)	7(78)	4(54)	6(34)	2(68)
Cocoa, drinking chocolate, etc	0(21) 6	0(28) 5	0(24) 11	0(23) 36	0(31) 20	0(27) 9	0(32) 3
Horlicks, Ovaltine	0(40) 13	0(45) 6	0(43) 19	0(33) 29	0(24) 17	0(47) 12	0(41) 8
Milk shakes	0(0) 0	0(0) 0	0(0) 0	0(330) 2	0(0) 0	0(0) 0	0(0) 0
Colas	0(84) 22	0(814) 13	0(830) 35	0(779) 91	0(185) 44	0(488) 24	0(749) 15
Fizzy drinks	396(598)	330(452)	336(541)	182(505)	310(518)	200(497)	285(641)
Other soft drinks	20(169) 14	0(394) 14	0(354) 38	0(897) 82	0(268) 62	0(241) 23	0(116) 13

Table 48 (Cont)

Food	One parent families			Two parent families			
	One child	Two or more children	All one parent families	One child	Two children	Three children	Four or more children
Alcoholic drinks:							
Beers and lagers	0(866) 9	0(0) 0	0(934) 10	0(1,033) 21	0(423) 16	0(559) 5	0(0) 0
Wines	0(141) 5	0(0) 0	0(125) 6	0(248) 14	0(148) 14	0(0) 0	0(87) 2
Spirits	0(25) 2	0(0) 0	0(25) 2	0(67) 4	0(60) 1	0(0) 0	0(0) 0
Other foods:							
Pickles and sauces	20(60)	11(42)	15(53)	16(49)	9(50)	0(61) 26	0(58) 16
Soups	0(554) 22	0(353) 8	0(501) 30	0(489) 98	116(203)	0(507) 26	0(484) 18
Number of children	49	31	80	207	131	58	37

Family composition

Table 49: *Foods consumed by boys aged 14/15 years (g/head/week)*

Food	Employment and benefits (benefits are also received by one-parent families)				
	Father unemployed	Father in employment	Family Income Supplement (FIS)	Supplementary Benefit (SB)	Neither FIS or SB
Number of children	69	363	15	68	444
Cereals:					
White bread	662(755)	592(661)	481(764)	647(677)	605(666)
Brown bread	0(155) 6	0(230) 74	0(140) 4	0(82) 8	0(225) 82
Wholemeal bread	0(195) 11	0(254) 82	0(443) 3	0(124) 6	0(235) 97
Other bread	0(376) 17	0(149) 90	0(25) 2	0(546) 16	0(161) 102
Total bread	(892)	(802)	(890)	(824)	(794)
Bran products	0(117) 3	0(245) 15	0(0) 0	0(0) 0	0(214) 19
Buns and pastries	0(115) 34	0(137) 173	111(142)	0(143) 32	0(133) 204
Cakes	80(117)	150(202)	107(133)	112(155)	136(202)
Biscuits	106(164)	164(201)	98(90)	131(175)	165(201)
Breakfast cereals	180(234)	222(257)	100(211)	194(267)	227(255)
Puddings, etc	288(308)	312(379)	268(369)	265(309)	292(373)
Icecream	0(125) 12	0(128) 133	0(90) 2	0(73) 13	0(134) 159
Rice	0(709) 12	0(231) 94	0(182) 2	0(531) 11	0(258) 108
Pasta	0(345) 23	0(276) 134	0(228) 3	0(240) 18	0(281) 160

Table 49 (Cont)

Food	Employment and benefits (benefits are also received by one-parent families)				
	Father unemployed	Father in employment	Family Income Supplement (FIS)	Supplementary Benefit (SB)	Neither FIS or SB
Milk and milk products:					
Cows milk, whole	1,539(1,592)	1,821(2,012)	1,321(1,518)	1,406(1,589)	1,766(1,976)
Skimmed, semi skimmed milk	0(1,776)	0(780)	0(0)	0(1,543)	0(963)
	2	7	0	3	9
Other milk	0(83)	0(141)	0(920)	0(69)	0(115)
	12	41	1	14	50
Yogurt	0(303)	0(253)	0(12)	0(198)	0(256)
	6	93	1	6	110
Cream	0(23)	0(38)	0(22)	0(27)	0(37)
	11	85	5	13	96
Cottage cheese	0(0)	0(0)	0(0)	0(0)	0(0)
	0	0	0	0	0
Cheese	88(142)	82(134)	31(102)	103(146)	82(136)
Eggs, egg dishes	107(170)	113(156)	156(141)	100(152)	113(160)
Fats and oils:					
Butter	21(61)	44(69)	36(64)	24(44)	40(67)
Margarine	0(87)	2(38)	14(51)	10(34)	2(42)
	33				
Low fat spread	0(0)	0(28)	0(63)	0(0)	0(9)
	0	6	2	0	4
Vegetable oils	0(5)	0(21)	0(18)	0(0)	0(19)
	1	15	4	0	13
Other fats and oils	0(102)	0(70)	0(0)	0(0)	0(69)
	2	19	0	0	21

Table 49 (Cont)

Food	Employment and benefits (benefits are also received by one-parent families)				
	Father unemployed	Father in employment	Family Income Supplement (FIS)	Supplementary Benefit (SB)	Neither FIS or SB
Carcase meats:					
Bacon and ham	32(57)	46(78)	48(63)	22(55)	46(76)
Beef and veal	0(248) 33	64(115)	0(205) 7	0(199) 31	56(114)
Mutton and lamb	0(287) 26	0(155) 124	0(145) 3	0(304) 20	0(163) 147
Pork	0(102) 19	0(131) 167	0(172) 6	0(98) 22	0(128) 183
Other meat:					
Chicken fried in breadcrumbs	0(0) 0	0(152) 5	0(127) 1	0(118) 2	0(130) 6
Poultry and game	74(91)	94(124)	76(100)	50(100)	90(120)
Liver	0(114) 12	0(112) 82	0(0) 0	0(148) 12	0(107) 97
Kidney	0(0) 0	0(57) 7	0(0) 0	0(136) 2	0(53) 8
Other offals	0(53) 3	0(60) 11	0(0) 0	0(0) 0	0(59) 14
Sausages	83(109)	103(142)	98(125)	90(109)	104(138)
Burgers	0(152) 33	32(70)	40(64)	42(69)	35(73)
Other meat products	412(473)	400(467)	372(461)	390(432)	405(476)

Table 49 (Cont)

Food	Employment and benefits (benefits are also received by one-parent families)				
	Father unemployed	Father in employment	Family Income Supplement (FIS)	Supplementary Benefit (SB)	Neither FIS or SB
Fish and fish products:					
Fish in batter or breadcrumbs	0(162)	0(150)	0(132)	0(155)	0(157)
	25	107	2	31	125
Fish fingers	0(99)	0(110)	0(0)	0(128)	0(111)
	18	90	0	21	105
Shellfish	0(49)	0(74)	0(60)	0(0)	0(70)
	2	61	1	0	19
Other fish	0(159)	0(106)	0(89)	0(117)	0(110)
	18	122	5	17	149
Sugar, sweets:					
Sugar	197(225)	183(200)	184(205)	196(208)	175(205)
Syrup and preserves	0(70)	0(73)	0(34)	0(48)	0(76)
	23	177	5	28	202
Chocolate	68(153)	108(170)	228(175)	86(157)	106(170)
Sweets	10(44)	12(72)	8(60)	19(49)	15(71)
Potatoes and potato products:					
Crisps, corn snacks, etc	28(61)	62(81)	50(66)	29(57)	57(85)
Chips	926(970)	597(729)	755(902)	917(974)	644(723)
Potatoes	433(544)	572(599)	412(424)	439(553)	560(601)

175

Table 49 (Cont)

Food	Employment and benefits (benefits are also received by one-parent families)				
	Father unemployed	Father in employment	Family Income Supplement (FIS)	Supplementary Benefit (SB)	Neither FIS or SB
Vegetables:					
Carrots	0(110) 30	30(56)	40(52)	0(167) 32	25(54)
Tomatoes	0(112) 15	0(105) 143	14(50)	0(92) 23	0(106) 158
Baked beans	220(244)	134(230)	258(311)	220(261)	140(226)
Peas	116(133)	77(106)	60(53)	118(146)	80(106)
Salad vegetables	0(42) 15	0(60) 135	0(64) 6	0(48) 20	0(60) 155
Other vegetables	110(175)	174(206)	111(123)	116(165)	154(209)
Fruit:					
Citrus fruit	0(171) 20	0(256) 134	0(177) 5	0(166) 15	0(245) 156
Apples and pears	0(251) 32	0(318) 175	0(344) 5	0(243) 29	0(315) 205
Other fresh fruit	0(190) 14	0(154) 115	0(197) 6	0(145) 9	0(154) 133
Other fruit	0(170) 16	0(166) 138	0(84) 6	0(161) 13	0(165) 156
Nuts:					
Nuts	0(51) 6	0(58) 34	0(71) 2	0(68) 7	0(59) 34
Peanut butter	0(76) 6	0(44) 25	0(52) 2	0(78) 4	0(45) 31

Table 49 (Cont)

Food	Employment and benefits (benefits are also received by one-parent families)				
	Father unemployed	Father in employment	Family Income Supplement (FIS)	Supplementary Benefit (SB)	Neither FIS or SB
Beverages:					
Fruit juices	0(269) 8	0(415) 102	0(330) 4	0(327) 8	0(425) 119
Tea	2,254(2,082)	1,385(1,672)	2,305(1,970)	1,778(1,703)	1,384(1,551)
Coffee	4(34)	4(63)	4(73)	0(28)	4(65)
Cocoa, drinking chocolate, etc.	0(22) 9	0(27) 57	0(24) 5	0(31) 11	0(25) 63
Horlicks, Ovaltine	0(46) 16	0(31) 50	0(42) 4	0(50) 20	0(31) 61
Milk shakes	0(0) 0	0(330) 2	0(0) 0	0(0) 0	0(322) 3
Colas	0(569) 20	0(692) 153	0(678) 3	0(739) 28	0(701) 176
Fizzy drinks	250(555)	250(527)	0(831)	379(525)	250(531)
Other soft drinks	0(423) 21	0(292) 162	0(565) 5	0(407) 21	0(304) 190
Alcoholic drinks:					
Beers and lagers	0(2,038) 1	0(727) 38	0(1,002) 2	0(341) 1	0(788) 47
Wines	0(0) 0	0(186) 30	0(0) 0	0(84) 3	0(189) 32
Spirits	0(0) 0	0(45) 3	0(0) 0	0(0) 0	0(56) 7

Table 49 (Cont)

Food	Employment and benefits (benefits are also received by one-parent families)				
	Father unemployed	Father in employment	Family Income Supplement (FIS)	Supplementary Benefit (SB)	Neither FIS or SB
Other foods:					
Pickles and sauces	0(80) 32	10(48)	10(45)	0(82) 32	11(47)
Soups	0(409) 30	0(464) 179	0(504) 7	0(434) 22	48(195)
Number of children	69	363	15	68	444

Table 50: *Food consumed by boys aged 14/15 years (g/head/week)*

Food	Type of lunch						
	Paid school meal	Free school meal	Paid school meal most days	Free school meal most days	Home	Packed lunch	Cafe
Number of children	86	50	58	25	119	105	68
Cereals:							
White bread	541(584)	614(746)	475(550)	526(598)	698(720)	694(788)	482(597)
Brown bread	0(115)	0(91)	0(195)	0(88)	0(211)	0(346)	0(57)
	15	7	12	3	25	27	5
Wholemeal bread	0(126)	0(163)	0(176)	0(422)	0(218)	0(320)	0(277)
	18	8	13	2	25	27	12
Other bread	0(240)	0(250)	0(111)	0(601)	0(286)	0(93)	0(160)
	20	12	11	6	26	30	15
Total bread	(688)	(842)	(647)	(785)	(872)	(989)	(689)
Bran products	0(100)	0(0)	0(19)	0(0)	0(116)	0(308)	0(3)
	3	0	2	0	3	10	1
Buns and pastries	33(82)	40(90)	48(54)	22(64)	0(150)	25(64)	0(95)
					50		24
Cakes	161(212)	142(220)	118(194)	170(216)	97(167)	173(202)	102(154)
Biscuits	169(189)	140(173)	135(203)	60(106)	148(195)	194(241)	150(185)
Breakfast cereals	239(253)	160(210)	220(253)	232(271)	222(267)	259(280)	170(220)
Puddings, etc	266(397)	279(362)	325(412)	334(381)	297(348)	282(373)	217(288)
Icecream	0(114)	0(91)	0(142)	0(95)	0(123)	0(132)	0(158)
	26	11	21	5	39	41	18
Rice	0(304)	0(186)	0(310)	0(1,057)	0(227)	0(223)	0(303)
	17	6	18	4	25	38	9
Pasta	0(307)	0(205)	0(179)	0(271)	0(336)	0(276)	0(235)
	33	16	21	7	47	39	14

Table 50 (Cont)

Food	Type of lunch						
	Paid school meal	Free school meal	Paid school meal most days	Free school meal most days	Home	Packed lunch	Cafe
Milk and milk products:							
Cows milk, whole	2,042(1,934)	1,092(1,390)	1,736(1,848)	1,406(1,656)	1,941(2,074)	1,766(2,110)	1,719(1,852)
Skimmed, semi skimmed milk	0(1,009) 4	0(2,443) 1	0(647) 3	0(748) 1	0(1,307) 2	0(0) 0	0(0) 0
Other milk	0(108) 8	0(80) 14	0(186) 11	0(30) 5	0(111) 12	0(139) 8	0(217) 8
Yogurt	0(298) 14	0(251) 10	0(284) 16	0(122) 3	0(283) 26	0(218) 34	0(269) 14
Cream	0(36) 26	0(26) 9	0(30) 11	0(16) 5	0(32) 25	0(40) 23	0(48) 13
Cottage cheese	0(0) 0	0(0) 0	0(0) 0	0(0) 0	0(0) 0	0(0) 0	0(0) 0
Cheese	131(179)	95(154)	42(115)	52(124)	87(123)	94(200)	44(103)
Eggs, egg dishes	94(132)	98(144)	98(162)	143(154)	115(156)	114(158)	156(205)
Fats and oils:							
Butter	38(61)	28(45)	53(70)	16(38)	50(72)	39(80)	14(36)
Margarine	0(53) 40	19(62)	0(60) 28	11(30)	0(92) 53	24(61)	7(28)
Low fat spread	0(0) 0	0(0) 0	0(0) 0	0(0) 0	0(18) 1	0(36) 4	0(0) 0
Vegetable oils	0(18) 3	0(5) 1	0(18) 2	0(0) 0	0(18) 2	0(27) 6	0(8) 2
Other fats and oils	0(69) 4	0(0) 0	0(4) 1	0(0) 0	0(32) 3	0(89) 8	0(86) 3

Table 50 (Cont)

Food	Type of lunch						
	Paid school meal	Free school meal	Paid school meal most days	Free school meal most days	Home	Packed lunch	Cafe
Carcase meats:							
Bacon and ham	34(63)	38(53)	51(72)	41(71)	30(68)	62(97)	62(72)
Beef and veal	70(108)	0(260) 24	72(114)	0(168) 10	0(256) 56	0(190) 51	104(123)
Mutton and lamb	0(130) 32	0(330) 13	0(158) 17	0(264) 9	0(195) 49	0(147) 25	0(157) 28
Pork	0(127) 39	0(116) 18	0(100) 29	0(109) 6	0(124) 44	0(115) 50	0(115) 22
Other meat:							
Chicken fried in breadcrumbs	0(0) 0	0(36) 1	0(0) 0	0(100) 3	0(137) 3	0(0) 0	0(0) 0
Poultry and game	80(100)	50(77)	83(103)	112(140)	84(115)	90(129)	98(140)
Liver	0(123) 11	0(140) 7	0(95) 5	0(23) 15	0(110) 27	0(103) 44	0(88) 8
Kidney	0(0) 0	0(3) 1	0(0) 0	0(2) 1	0(77) 3	0(18) 3	0(16) 1
Other offals	0(53) 3	0(39) 2	0(0) 0	0(0) 0	0(60) 5	0(0) 0	0(76) 4
Sausages	118(142)	72(102)	110(138)	142(127)	107(153)	100(124)	100(120)
Burgers	32(76)	52(84)	0(167) 26	75(98)	23(59)	40(85)	0(116) 30
Other meat products	400(475)	460(519)	400(464)	372(371)	404(454)	371(433)	529(558)

Table 50 (Cont)

Food	Type of lunch						
	Paid school meal	Free school meal	Paid school meal most days	Free school meal most days	Home	Packed lunch	Cafe
Fish and fish products:							
Fish in batter or breadcrumbs	0(141) 28	0(146) 24	0(167) 16	0(195) 9	0(159) 36	0(136) 20	0(168) 22
Fish fingers	0(97) 19	0(99) 11	0(117) 17	0(122) 7	0(122) 35	0(122) 22	0(123) 15
Shellfish	0(96) 5	0(0) 0	0(42) 2	0(60) 1	0(43) 3	0(59) 7	0(95) 2
Other fish	0(115) 26	0(50) 15	0(145) 19	0(173) 8	0(109) 30	0(101) 46	0(97) 22
Sugar, sweets:							
Sugar	184(198)	153(184)	158(202)	146(193)	204(245)	157(180)	168(209)
Syrup and preserves	3(31)	0(55) 23	0(70) 26	0(45) 8	0(68) 47	12(45)	0(92) 29
Chocolate	83(201)	42(145)	119(188)	68(132)	97(133)	108(149)	188(236)
Sweets	6(77)	30(70)	22(75)	10(39)	14(69)	0(106) 49	20(81)
Potatoes and potato products:							
Crisps, corn snacks, etc	31(62)	25(50)	55(75)	26(50)	56(83)	105(105)	75(102)
Chips	851(900)	1,102(1,079)	951(946)	840(948)	434(568)	340(400)	1,050(1,015)
Potatoes	600(659)	466(586)	439(542)	597(569)	572(598)	584(649)	360(442)

Table 50 (Cont)

Food	Type of lunch						
	Paid school meal	Free school meal	Paid school meal most days	Free school meal most days	Home	Packed lunch	Cafe
Vegetables:							
Carrots	33(52) 24	0(97) 24	32(52)	0(147) 9	29(51)	41(57)	0(127) 28
Tomatoes	0(108) 30	0(104) 17	0(108) 22	0(65) 10	0(112) 40	0(104) 41	0(95) 28
Baked beans	222(293)	228(325)	205(280)	230(251)	130(227)	106(142)	92(194)
Peas	86(120)	100(131)	76(94)	100(114)	87(116)	82(106)	83(100)
Salad vegetables	0(57) 30	0(61) 16	0(60) 14	0(61) 8	0(45) 37	0(73) 49	0(53) 26
Other vegetables	145(227)	172(205)	151(170)	143(146)	122(188)	202(244)	133(164)
Fruit:							
Citrus fruit	0(256) 27	0(178) 15	0(361) 26	0(144) 6	0(195) 40	0(195) 49	0(244) 14
Apples and pears	69(144)	0(199) 16	0(277) 28	0(318) 8	0(263) 50	174(253)	0(294) 29
Other fresh fruit	0(133) 24	0(137) 8	0(159) 18	0(205) 3	0(165) 32	0(167) 38	0(135) 22
Other fruit	0(151) 38	0(139) 12	0(173) 14	0(198) 5	0(190) 31	0(185) 46	0(109) 28
Nuts:							
Nuts	0(37) 8	0(79) 8	0(66) 4	0(0) 0	0(68) 7	0(64) 10	0(46) 6
Peanut butter	0(24) 7	0(31) 2	0(33) 2	0(96) 1	0(36) 6	0(66) 17	0(0) 0

Table 50 (Cont)

Food	Type of lunch						
	Paid school meal	Free school meal	Paid school meal most days	Free school meal most days	Home	Packed lunch	Cafe
Beverages:							
Fruit juices	0(607) / 22	0(256) / 9	0(455) / 20	0(479) / 4	0(196) / 18	0(471) / 37	0(337) / 18
Tea	916(1,552)	1,558(1,717)	99(1,430)	1,778(1,942)	2,130(2,270)	1,304(1,547)	1,584(1,729)
Coffee	5(56) / 21	0(82) / 21	6(33)	6(25)	8(70)	0(200) / 50	4(22)
Cocoa, drinking chocolate, etc	0(36) / 15	0(30) / 10	0(32) / 10	0(22) / 2	0(24) / 18	0(15) / 16	0(20) / 5
Horlicks, Ovaltine	0(43) / 20	0(51) / 17	0(29) / 17	0(37) / 9	0(21) / 9	0(13) / 6	0(34) / 7
Milk shakes	0(0) / 0	0(0) / 0	0(0) / 0	0(0) / 0	0(3) / 1	0(5) / 1	0(4) / 1
Colas	0(643) / 28	0(773) / 17	201(392)	0(744) / 10	0(682) / 43	0(712) / 42	180(377)
Fizzy drinks	274(414)	330(544)	328(618)	271(402)	223(595)	250(435)	200(645)
Other soft drinks	0(273) / 36	0(292) / 21	0(249) / 27	0(231) / 6	0(377) / 39	40(167)	0(396) / 31
Alcoholic drinks:							
Beers and lagers	0(547) / 10	0(556) / 2	0(670) / 11	0(950) / 2	0(517) / 12	0(1,223) / 10	0(1,183) / 2
Wines	0(155) / 7	0(103) / 3	0(172) / 4	0(59) / 2	0(192) / 4	0(273) / 9	0(130) / 4
Spirits	0(0) / 0	0(0) / 0	0(83) / 3	0(0) / 0	0(28) / 2	0(0) / 0	0(35) / 1

Table 50 (Cont)

Food	Type of lunch						
	Paid school meal	Free school meal	Paid school meal most days	Free school meal most days	Home	Packed lunch	Cafe
Other foods:							
Pickles and sauces	9(44)	0(90) 23	0(101) 29	12(45)	6(44)	16(51)	12(47)
Soups	0(414) 40	0(316) 12	0(426) 28	0(535) 10	225(363)	0(373) 38	180(220)
Number of children	86	50	58	25	119	105	68

185

Table 51: *Foods consumed by boys aged 14/15 years (g/head/week)*

Food	Type of school meal (excludes those not taking a school meal)		
	Cafeteria	Fixed price	Other
Number of children	182	30	4
Cereals:			
White bread	544(611)	519(586)	(*)
Brown bread	0(138)	0(100)	(*)
	31	5	
Wholemeal bread	0(168)	0(114)	(*)
	33	4	
Other bread	0(236)	0(409)	(*)
	42	7	
Total bread	(719)	(700)	(*)
Bran products	0(45)	0(114)	(*)
	4	1	
Buns and pastries	22(66)	90(119)	(*)
Cakes	156(219)	138(163)	(*)
Biscuits	140(189)	78(139)	(*)
Breakfast cereals	220(255)	194(197)	(*)
Puddings, etc	290(366)	442(552)	(*)
Icecream	0(125)	0(98)	(*)
	48	12	
Rice	0(410)	0(121)	(*)
	37	7	
Pasta	0(237)	0(329)	(*)
	64	9	
Milk and milk products:			
Cows milk, whole	1,590(1,782)	1,303(1,575)	(*)
Skimmed, semi skimmed milk	0(1,049)	0(893)	(*)
	7	2	
Other milk	0(118)	0(59)	(*)
	32	5	
Yogurt	0(271)	0(240)	(*)
	41	2	
Cream	0(73)	0(22)	(*)
	41	11	
Cottage cheese	0(0)	0(0)	(*)
	0	0	
Cheese	101(157)	79(120)	(*)
Eggs, egg dishes	92(133)	151(192)	(*)
Fats and oils:			
Butter	38(59)	26(47)	(*)
Margarine	0(68)	18(31)	(*)
	90		
Low fat spread	0(0)	0(0)	(*)
	0	0	
Vegetable oils	0(13)	0(0)	(*)
	5	0	
Other fats and oils	0(61)	0(66)	(*)
	5	2	

Table 51 (Cont)

Food	Type of school meal (excludes those not taking a school meal)		
	Cafeteria	Fixed price	Other
Carcase meat:			
Bacon and ham	40(61)	57(75)	(*)
Beef and veal	48(101)	61(170)	(*)
Mutton and lamb	0(191)	0(187)	(*)
	59	11	
Pork	0(116)	0(113)	(*)
	77	15	
Other meat:			
Chicken fried in breadcrumbs	0(58)	0(127)	(*)
	6	1	
Poultry and game	80(99)	68(110)	(*)
Liver	0(19)	0(8)	(*)
	24	4	
Kidney	0(0)	0(0)	(*)
	0	0	
Other offals	0(45)	0(60)	(*)
	4	1	
Sausages	104(130)	121(140)	(*)
Burgers	38(79)	46(80)	(*)
Other meat products	400(473)	374(418)	(*)
Fish and fish products:			
Fish in batter or breadcrumbs	0(146)	0(158)	(*)
	61	11	
Fish fingers	0(102)	0(101)	(*)
	46	7	
Shellfish	0(79)	0(160)	(*)
	8	1	
Other fish	0(110)	0(165)	(*)
	58	10	
Sugar, sweets:			
Sugar	169(193)	197(210)	(*)
Syrup and preserves	0(60)	0(66)	(*)
	88	12	
Chocolate	85(176)	114(203)	(*)
Sweets	21(77)	17(39)	(*)
Potatoes and potato products:			
Crisps, corn snacks, etc	32(62)	28(63)	(*)
Chips	948(981)	766(784)	(*)
Potatoes	492(592)	615(698)	(*)
Vegetables:			
Carrots	22(50)	0(118)	(*)
		6	
Tomatoes	0(102)	0(101)	(*)
	64	14	
Baked beans	220(291)	285(290)	(*)
Peas	86(113)	129(125)	(*)
Salad vegetables	0(58)	0(59)	(*)
	59	7	
Other vegetables	143(195)	193(223)	(*)

187

Table 51 (Cont)

Food	Type of school meal (excludes those not taking a school meal)		
	Cafeteria	Fixed price	Other
Fruit:			
Citrus fruit	0(264)	0(283)	(*)
	64	10	
Apples and pears	0(285)	96(120)	(*)
	76		
Other fresh fruit	0(114)	0(133)	(*)
	44	9	
Other fruit	0(160)	0(151)	(*)
	54	11	
Nuts:			
Nuts	0(66)	0(20)	(*)
	18	3	
Peanut butter	0(46)	0(17)	(*)
	7	5	
Beverages:			
Fruit juices	0(495)	0(465)	(*)
	46	8	
Tea	916(1,507)	2,072(2,024)	(*)
Coffee	5(37)	2(76)	(*)
Cocoa, drinking chocolate, etc	0(32)	0(44)	(*)
	35	3	
Horlicks, Ovaltine	0(38)	10(25)	(*)
	46		
Milk shakes	0(0)	0(0)	(*)
	0	0	
Colas	0(736)	0(536)	(*)
	75	9	
Fizzy drinks	274(496)	434(502)	(*)
Other soft drinks	0(253)	0(408)	(*)
	78	10	
Alcoholic drinks:			
Beers and lagers	0(636)	0(679)	(*)
	24	2	
Wines	0(142)	0(123)	(*)
	10	4	
Spirits	0(72)	0(0)	(*)
	4	0	
Other foods:			
Pickles and sauces	10(48)	0(68)	(*)
		14	
Soups	0(399)	0(521)	(*)
	77	13	
Number of children	182	30	4

Table 52: *Foods consumed by girls aged 14/15 years (g/head/week)*

Food	National median	I	II	IIInm	IIIm	IV	V
			Social class (excludes unemployed and one parent families)				
Number of children	461	25	70	44	94	64	15
Cereals:							
White bread	433(480)	338(381)	399(436)	381(512)	482(521)	432(460)	434(443)
Brown bread	0(159) 72	0(361) 8	0(84) 17	0(159) 7	0(133) 12	0(210) 7	0(0) 0
Wholemeal bread	0(214) 101	0(244) 8	0(283) 29	0(146) 6	0(202) 20	0(91) 8	0(145) 5
Other bread	0(144) 130	0(88) 11	0(117) 21	0(104) 21	0(83) 18	0(159) 17	0(185) 3
Total bread	(595)	(623)	(610)	(606)	(597)	(556)	(693)
Bran products	0(124) 19	0(237) 1	0(114) 6	0(143) 2	0(69) 3	0(66) 5	0(0) 0
Buns and pastries	31(68)	64(92)	0(136) 30	0(118) 18	40(69)	34(62)	50(92)
Cakes	118(163)	229(250)	160(222)	146(160)	92(146)	92(126)	66(91)
Biscuits	118(150)	143(152)	104(124)	118(156)	103(156)	118(153)	88(108)
Breakfast cereals	72(122)	70(134)	110(134)	80(118)	72(124)	64(113)	69(96)
Puddings, etc	220(265)	318(346)	246(275)	200(252)	240(301)	156(223)	130(166)
Icecream	0(101) 147	0(42) 6	0(101) 31	0(75) 13	0(107) 25	0(93) 21	0(77) 5
Rice	0(260) 116	0(154) 6	0(243) 23	0(239) 13	0(376) 19	0(239) 15	0(178) 4
Pasta	0(222) 168	12(211)	0(243) 20	2(92)	0(203) 33	0(268) 26	0(171) 6

Table 52 (Cont)

Food	Social class (excludes unemployed and one parent families)						
	National median	I	II	IIInm	IIIm	IV	V
Milk and milk products:							
Cows milk, whole	1,153(1,296)	1,204(1,283)	1,350(1,449)	1,133(1,341)	1,385(1,495)	922(1,140)	1,077(1,120)
Skimmed, semi skimmed milk	0(594)	0(0)	0(693)	0(1,026)	0(575)	0(764)	0(0)
	17	0	2	1	2	1	0
Other milk	0(86)	0(0)	0(65)	0(25)	0(91)	0(203)	0(443)
	50	0	9	8	10	5	1
Yogurt	0(267)	0(269)	0(243)	0(357)	0(252)	0(296)	0(212)
	123	1	22	10	23	22	2
Cream	0(43)	0(40)	0(54)	0(39)	0(53)	0(29)	0(16)
	116	11	28	12	16	14	3
Cottage cheese	0(76)	0(0)	0(45)	0(0)	0(28)	0(0)	0(0)
	15	0	6	0	4	0	0
Cheese	71(106)	76(106)	114(146)	67(105)	64(95)	60(95)	40(102)
Eggs, egg dishes	95(118)	61(95)	60(99)	103(101)	82(112)	88(117)	96(156)
Fats and oils:							
Butter	25(45)	34(62)	40(56)	18(46)	76(50)	20(37)	39(37)
Margarine	11(35)	0(53)	0(75)	21(46)	10(38)	10(28)	17(35)
Low fat spread	0(41)	0(6)	0(17)	0(0)	0(41)	0(0)	0(0)
	9	2	1	0	3	0	0
Vegetable oils	0(16)	0(17)	0(16)	0(8)	0(26)	0(0)	0(0)
	18	2	3	2	4	0	0
Other fats and oils	0(41)	0(0)	0(49)	0(58)	0(55)	0(25)	0(0)
	27	0	11	3	3	2	0

Table 52 (Cont)

Food		Social class (excludes unemployed and one parent families)					
	National median	I	II	IIInm	IIIm	IV	V
Carcase meats:							
Bacon and ham	39(58)	68(85)	50(66)	50(59)	48(63)	38(56)	0(139) 7
Beef and veal	23(79)	56(83)	0(165) 33	27(78)	56(94)	44(89)	0(123) 5
Mutton and lamb	0(36) 142	0(133) 9	0(101) 16	0(101) 13	0(122) 24	0(155) 22	0(131) 3
Pork	0(119) 202	0(119) 9	0(141) 33	0(92) 18	0(133) 43	0(109) 30	0(104) 7
Other meats:							
Chicken fried in breadcrumbs	0(112) 10	0(0) 0	0(90) 1	0(0) 0	0(106) 3	0(95) 2	0(0) 0
Poultry and game	65(104)	80(128)	106(139)	60(96)	70(109)	65(96)	32(123)
Liver	0(184) 95	0(98) 9	0(71) 18	0(40) 10	0(78) 20	0(69) 9	0(241) 2
Kidney	0(71) 13	0(0) 0	0(0) 0	0(0) 0	0(0) 0	0(0) 0	0(0) 0
Other offals	0(21) 3	0(86) 2	0(0) 0	0(67) 3	0(38) 3	0(89) 3	0(0) 0
Sausages	50(80)	0(173) 8	40(70)	46(50)	50(69)	54(110)	51(78)
Burgers	0(105) 189	0(126) 8	0(108) 24	0(106) 10	0(109) 39	0(91) 27	0(79) 4
Other meat products	312(362)	294(373)	316(330)	261(297)	346(374)	296(343)	305(355)

191

Table 52 (Cont)

Food	National median	Social class (excludes unemployed and one parent families)					
		I	II	IIInm	IIIm	IV	V
Fish in fish products:							
Fish in batter or breadcrumbs	0(135) 141	0(147) 5	0(131) 17	0(99) 14	0(149) 23	0(144) 29	0(191) 4
Fish fingers	0(100) 123	0(100) 7	0(103) 16	0(64) 14	0(113) 27	0(86) 15	0(71) 6
Shellfish	0(38) 11	0(0) 0	0(38) 3	0(26) 2	0(51) 3	0(30) 2	0(0) 0
Other fish	0(79) 148	0(60) 11	0(93) 20	0(76) 13	0(96) 31	0(85) 21	0(111) 3
Sugar, sweets:							
Sugar	85(112)	5(53)	46(65)	83(115)	105(136)	86(109)	81(107)
Syrup and preserves	0(47) 200	21(27) 11	14(32)	0(55) 21	0(49) 36	0(40) 24	0(27) 5
Chocolate	72(119)	76(87)	68(127)	84(97)	94(116)	113(177)	68(138)
Sweets	18(57)	0(33)	2(44)	25(55)	30(59)	10(66)	40(74)
Potatoes and potato products:							
Crisps, corn snacks, etc	75(95)	30(61)	78(85)	50(85)	83(103)	100(127)	108(121)
Chips	442(550)	250(303)	294(432)	472(581)	486(565)	500(522)	381(494)
Potatoes	430(492)	458(490)	426(484)	385(445)	490(516)	426(496)	411(417)

Table 52 (Cont)

Food	National median	Social class (excludes unemployed and one parent families)					
		I	II	IIInm	IIIm	IV	V
Vegetables:							
Carrots	24(47)	60(97)	24(39)	25(43)	23(48)	0(101) 27	0(72) 7
Tomatoes	0(113) 216	88(86)	16(53)	0(88) 19	0(114) 42	0(112) 30	0(66) 6
Baked beans	68(143)	5(210)	57(116)	0(326) 19	78(141)	0(233) 31	160(218)
Peas	66(92)	90(96)	44(72)	34(59)	96(105)	42(82)	52(99)
Salad vegetables	0(66) 207	25(64)	17(44)	0(46) 18	0(54) 41	0(65) 25	4(19)
Other vegetables	175(211)	336(439)	187(221)	167(201)	180(207)	150(177)	109(198)
Fruit:							
Citrus fruit	0(232) 201	0(252) 10	102(134)	0(168) 18	0(242) 40	0(248) 25	18(79)
Apples and pears	90(165)	0(377) 12	109(180)	116(156)	0(343) 46	0(284) 42	114(173)
Other fresh fruit	0(170) 116	0(95) 11	0(165) 19	0(118) 10	0(173) 14	0(201) 17	0(128) 4
Other fruit	0(112) 176	10(57)	38(63)	0(63) 17	0(126) 28	0(115) 25	0(132) 4
Nuts:							
Nuts	0(34) 44	0(34) 1	0(43) 8	0(43) 3	0(31) 9	0(14) 5	0(115) 2
Peanut butter	0(37) 40	0(87) 3	0(27) 9	0(34) 4	0(23) 7	0(33) 3	0(0) 0

Table 52 (Cont)

Food	National median	Social class (excludes unemployed and one parent families)					
		I	II	IIInm	IIIm	IV	V
Beverages:							
Fruit juices	0(376) / 186	106(252) / 2	4(220) / 17	0(260) / 22	0(317) / 39	0(475) / 22	0(210) / 7
Tea	1,021(1,399)	1,153(1,400)	272(883)	1,369(1,690)	1,351(1,485)	880(1,405)	400(1,029)
Coffee	4(46)	16(160)	4(62)	2(37)	7(36)	7(23)	0(16) / 7
Cocoa, drinking chocolate, etc.	0(27) / 96	0(25) / 2	0(24) / 17	0(20) / 12	0(31) / 18	0(32) / 13	0(34) / 2
Horlicks, ovaltine	0(25) / 83	0(49) / 3	0(23) / 12	0(25) / 7	0(21) / 18	0(23) / 9	0(28) / 2
Milk shakes	0(300) / 1	0(0) / 0	0(300) / 1	0(0) / 0	0(0) / 0	0(0) / 0	0(0) / 0
Colas	0(612) / 197	0(422) / 11	0(719) / 26	0(759) / 13	0(601) / 44	50(410)	0(744) / 7
Fizzy drinks	280(502) / 187	358(569)	244(473)	200(590)	330(502)	200(364)	526(580)
Other soft drinks	0(238) / 187	0(286) / 5	0(249) / 31	0(257) / 14	0(222) / 38	0(279) / 26	0(157) / 6
Alcoholic drinks:							
Beers and lagers	0(354) / 35	0(436) / 3	0(165) / 16	0(919) / 4	0(281) / 6	0(357) / 2	0(570) / 1
Wines	0(247) / 33	0(0) / 0	0(145) / 9	0(100) / 2	0(312) / 9	0(234) / 4	0(0) / 0
Spirits	0(49) / 9	0(44) / 1	0(19) / 4	0(0) / 0	0(147) / 2	0(0) / 0	0(30) / 1

Table 52 (Cont)

Food	Social class (excludes unemployed and one parent families)						
	National median	I	II	IIInm	IIIm	IV	V
Other foods:							
Pickles and sauces	12(40)	35(53)	30(62)	0(102) 17	10(35)	10(36)	0(49) 6
Soups	49(191)	130(152)	49(157)	0(407) 20	74(215)	0(390) 30	59(227)
Number of children	461	25	70	44	94	64	15

195

Table 53: *Foods consumed by girls aged 14/15 years (g/head/week)*

Food	Region			
	Scotland	London and SE	North	Rest of GB
Number of children	44	129	122	164
Cereals:				
White bread	503(533)	384(426)	432(479)	470(515)
Brown bread	0(91)	0(147)	0(151)	0(200)
	5	32	15	20
Wholemeal bread	0(66)	0(200)	0(244)	0(217)
	4	33	30	35
Other bread	0(98)	0(194)	0(165)	0(91)
	8	39	39	44
Total bread	(568)	(566)	(606)	(610)
Bran products	0(0)	0(128)	0(102)	0(141)
	0	6	6	7
Buns and pastries	0(69)	24(73)	50(81)	17(66)
	17			
Cakes	99(123)	134(164)	109(148)	122(184)
Biscuits	147(194)	122(158)	107(136)	119(143)
Breakfast cereals	54(77)	69(130)	71(128)	93(124)
Puddings, etc	341(346)	204(257)	224(249)	208(264)
Icecream	0(87)	0(133)	0(85)	0(93)
	20	39	26	52
Rice	0(217)	0(346)	0(198)	0(217)
	11	43	26	36
Pasta	0(226)	0(209)	0(252)	0(211)
	17	54	43	54

Table 53 (Cont)

Food	Region			
	Scotland	London and SE	North	Rest of GB
Milk and milk products:				
Cows milk, whole	954(1,370)	1,084(1,184)	1,112(1,261)	1,228(1,392)
Skimmed, semi skimmed milk	0(335)	0(658)	0(458)	0(402)
	1	6	6	3
Other milk	0(52)	0(93)	0(73)	0(99)
	4	18	13	15
Yogurt	0(243)	0(276)	0(254)	0(277)
	9	23	39	52
Cream	0(37)	0(47)	0(59)	0(31)
	10	28	32	46
Cottage cheese	0(0)	0(392)	0(54)	0(32)
	0	2	6	7
Cheese	91(138)	64(101)	57(88)	94(115)
Eggs, egg dishes	108(125)	81(99)	118(147)	61(109)
Fats and oils:				
Butter	22(46)	36(54)	11(30)	33(50)
Margarine	20(34)	0(50)	25(43)	10(39)
		62		
Low fat spread	0(0)	0(63)	0(6)	0(19)
	0	5	2	2
Vegetables oils	0(0)	0(13)	0(15)	0(20)
	0	7	6	5
Other fats and oils	0(0)	0(43)	0(21)	0(52)
	0	8	7	11

Table 53 (Cont)

Food	Region			
	Scotland	London and SE	North	Rest of GB
Carcase meats:				
Bacon and ham	66(68)	42(56)	33(55)	39(60)
Beef and veal	116(112)	62(88)	12(78)	0(151) 71
Mutton and lamb	0(83) 4	0(133) 41	0(117) 47	0(160) 50
Pork	0(103) 17	0(137) 58	0(104) 53	0(119) 75
Other meat:				
Chicken fried in breadcrumbs	0(0) 0	0(116) 6	0(127) 1	0(97) 3
Poultry and game	74(98)	109(139)	53(82)	60(95)
Liver	0(106) 3	0(83) 29	0(96) 26	0(74) 36
Kidney	0(0) 0	0(20) 3	0(0) 0	0(0) 0
Other offals	0(47) 5	0(78) 3	0(78) 2	0(89) 3
Sausages	85(117)	57(87)	44(70)	49(74)
Burgers	0(118) 12	0(105) 62	0(111) 59	0(96) 56
Other meat products	220(272)	294(339)	371(401)	328(372)

Table 53 (Cont)

Food	Region			
	Scotland	London and SE	North	Rest of GB
Fish and fish products:				
Fish in batter or breadcrumbs	60(80)	0(148) 26	0(133) 56	0(116) 38
Fish fingers	0(80) 7	0(112) 34	0(95) 39	0(97) 43
Shellfish	0(0) 0	0(39) 7	0(0) 0	0(41) 3
Other fish	0(18) 7	0(30) 42	0(24) 46	0(76) 53
Sugar, sweets:				
Sugar	98(109)	85(103)	85(114)	87(117)
Syrup and preserves	0(64) 21	0(44) 60	0(39) 51	0(49) 69
Chocolate	166(188)	72(119)	84(128)	58(94)
Sweets	75(129)	12(40)	36(71)	3(42)
Potatoes and potato products:				
Crisps, corn snacks, etc	95(127)	75(97)	69(91)	78(90)
Chips	419(575)	316(464)	582(633)	436(547)
Potatoes	340(385)	361(510)	407(454)	460(536)

Table 53 (Cont)

Food	Region			
	Scotland	London and SE	North	Rest of GB
Vegetables:				
Carrots	0(57) 9	0(80) 59	50(60)	25(53)
Tomatoes	0(101) 17	10(52)	0(101) 60	0(137) 73
Baked beans	73(104)	61(113)	46(143)	86(176)
Peas	30(47)	72(96)	66(95)	70(98)
Salad vegetables	0(52) 15	5(39)	0(63) 51	0(63) 72
Other vegetables	92(125)	167(240)	184(211)	192(211)
Fruit:				
Citrus fruit	0(166) 16	0(224) 65	0(231) 51	0(254) 70
Apples and pears	116(144)	72(190)	83(124)	88(182)
Other fresh fruit	0(185) 19	0(164) 32	0(187) 25	0(156) 41
Other fruit	60(73)	0(112) 54	0(108) 48	0(110) 50
Nuts:				
Nuts	0(25) 4	0(43) 10	0(38) 12	0(27) 18
Peanut butter	0(87) 2	0(23) 18	0(41) 8	0(45) 12

Table 53 (Cont)

Food	Region			
	Scotland	London and SE	North	Rest of GB
Beverages:				
Fruit juices	0(348) 13	41(249)	0(253) 41	0(360) 64
Tea	1,868(1,855)	1,042(1,321)	710(1,487)	842(1,279)
Coffee	6(83)	2(54)	7(54)	4(24)
Cocoa, drinking chocolate, etc.	0(62) 8	0(25) 28	0(22) 22	0(24) 37
Horlicks, Ovaltine	0(16) 4	0(23) 26	0(26) 25	0(26) 27
Milk shakes	0(0) 0	0(0) 0	0(0) 0	0(300) 1
Colas	400(751)	0(609) 63	0(500) 40	0(509) 62
Fizzy drinks	330(545)	200(377)	438(667)	200(464)
Other soft drinks	0(410) 19	0(293) 57	0(155) 41	0(195) 71
Alcoholic drinks:				
Beers and lagers	0(0) 0	0(234) 10	0(451) 12	0(351) 13
Wines	0(0) 0	0(223) 13	0(107) 6	0(317) 13
Spirits	0(0) 0	0(45) 4	0(105) 2	0(24) 3

Table 53 (Cont)

Food	Region			
	Scotland	London and SE	North	Rest of GB
Other foods:				
Pickles and sauces	8(33)	20(48)	10(37)	10(37)
Soups	306(463)	0(319)	78(199)	0(344)
		58		74
Number of children	42	129	122	164

202

Table 54: *Foods consumed by girls aged 14/15 years (g/head/week)*

	Family composition						
	One parent families			Two parent families			
Food	One child	Two or more children	All one parent families	One child	Two children	Three children	Four or more children
Number of children	38	33	75	159	142	52	35
Cereals:							
White bread	384(425)	442(522)	430(458)	432(479)	372(451)	499(528)	566(561)
Brown bread	0(106)	0(151)	0(124)	0(158)	0(172)	0(213)	0(49)
	5	3	9	28	24	5	1
Wholemeal bread	0(177)	0(165)	0(172)	0(186)	0(210)	0(372)	0(187)
	6	5	11	30	43	10	7
Other bread	0(54)	0(109)	0(76)	0(284)	0(107)	0(83)	0(163)
	9	7	19	52	36	14	11
Total bread	(483)	(586)	(518)	(606)	(576)	(647)	(650)
Bran products	0(0)	0(0)	0(141)	0(75)	0(143)	0(0)	0(203)
	0	0	1	8	8	0	1
Buns and pastries	38(72)	0(145)	17(70)	40(73)	29(64)	54(73)	0(140)
		14					16
Cakes	93(130)	152(160)	114(146)	108(163)	112(173)	150(178)	172(136)
Biscuits	132(151)	122(167)	126(159)	114(141)	111(147)	164(146)	112(121)
Breakfast cereals	43(141)	68(110)	61(132)	59(115)	93(130)	88(151)	74(113)
Puddings, etc	196(224)	177(239)	204(231)	220(281)	246(271)	185(254)	231(257)
Icecream	0(97)	0(106)	0(102)	0(87)	0(87)	0(130)	0(79)
	11	12	23	51	47	13	13
Rice	0(250)	0(197)	0(227)	0(259)	0(228)	0(226)	0(569)
	6	10	18	73	41	16	8
Pasta	0(285)	0(236)	0(258)	0(234)	0(202)	0(202)	0(209)
	14	10	25	46	61	24	14

Table 54 (Cont)

Food	Family composition						
	One parent families			Two parent families			
	One child	Two or more children	All one parent families	One child	Two children	Three children	Four or more children
Milk and milk products:							
Cows milk, whole	1,167(1,281)	1,063(1,186)	1,135(1,280)	1,234(1,365)	1,161(1,353)	1,051(1,186)	911(1,034)
Skimmed, semi skimmed milk	0(0) 0	0(664) 5	0(582) 5	0(655) 5	0(491) 4	0(0) 0	0(773) 2
Other milk	0(38) 3	0(147) 2	0(42) 6	0(78) 22	0(141) 14	0(62) 7	0(18) 2
Yogurt	0(250) 8	0(381) 8	0(315) 15	0(268) 47	0(300) 36	0(201) 17	0(164) 9
Cream	0(38) 7	0(52) 7	0(49) 17	0(29) 47	0(618) 41	0(36) 16	0(26) 7
Cottage cheese	0(0) 0	0(267) 2	0(267) 2	0(36) 5	0(85) 4	0(58) 3	0(20) 1
Cheese	28(72)	62(128)	40(95)	76(110)	76(105)	56(94)	86(122)
Eggs, egg dishes	70(111)	63(114)	63(108)	92(117)	100(120)	81(100)	113(145)
Fats and oils:							
Butter	34(46)	37(49)	30(45)	18(43)	31(48)	23(43)	11(47)
Margarine	12(26)	8(33)	12(30)	10(31)	10(49)	11(42)	28(41)
Low fat spread	0(54) 2	0(0) 0	0(70) 3	0(35) 2	0(17) 3	0(0) 0	0(0) 0
Vegetable oils	0(7) 2	0(0) 0	0(7) 3	0(22) 4	0(16) 8	0(9) 3	0(0) 0
Other fats and oils	0(11) 2	0(73) 4	0(55) 5	0(13) 6	0(39) 12	0(54) 4	0(26) 2

Table 54 (Cont)

Family composition

Food	One parent families			Two parent families			
	One child	Two or more children	All one parent families	One child	Two children	Three children	Four or more children
Carcase meats:							
Bacon and ham	45(68)	41(50)	41(57)	32(58)	39(60)	62(64)	10(40)
Beef and veal	22(89)	0(189)	20(88)	36(77)	70(88)	0(158)	0(113)
		15				23	14
Mutton and lamb	0(116)	0(110)	0(113)	0(127)	0(129)	0(126)	0(230)
	10	10	20	49	43	16	14
Pork	0(127)	0(106)	0(117)	0(121)	0(120)	25(62)	34(54)
	16	14	30	68	60		
Other meat:							
Chicken fried in breadcrumbs	0(134)	0(0)	0(139)	0(106)	0(100)	0(82)	0(0)
	3	0	3	1	2	1	0
Poultry and game	41(78)	8(86)	7(78)	67(113)	73(107)	92(96)	65(106)
Liver	0(82)	0(93)	0(87)	0(85)	0(84)	0(19)	0(85)
	5	4	9	34	33	18	7
Kidney	0(0)	0(0)	0(0)	0(0)	0(0)	0(0)	0(0)
Other offals	0(0)	0(0)	0(0)	0(69)	0(78)	0(0)	0(0)
	0	0	0	7	5	0	0
Sausages	53(99)	48(79)	50(86)	46(78)	55(80)	76(90)	33(60)
Burgers	0(114)	68(73)	36(68)	0(95)	0(116)	0(85)	0(101)
				62	53	18	17
Other meat products	347(441)	377(373)	397(415)	334(383)	246(308)	320(368)	346(375)

Table 54 (Cont)

Food	Family composition						
	One parent families			Two parent families			
	One child	Two or more children	All one parent families	One child	Two children	Three children	Four or more children
Fish and fish products:							
Fish in batter breadcrumbs	0(145) 10	0(104) 7	0(128) 21	0(130) 57	0(133) 43	0(99) 14	0(148) 10
Fish fingers	0(107) 10	0(134) 8	0(116) 21	0(106) 48	0(92) 36	0(73) 12	0(88) 8
Shellfish	0(0) 0	0(30) 1	0(30) 1	0(46) 5	0(30) 4	0(0) 0	0(0) 0
Other fish	0(78) 12	0(46) 7	0(77) 21	0(78) 50	0(79) 47	0(86) 16	0(71) 17
Sugar, sweets:							
Sugar	118(138) 16	55(95)	107(125)	85(113)	72(99)	119(121)	85(134)
Syrup and preserves	0(42) 16	0(37) 11	0(116) 30	0(43) 67	0(43) 67	0(65) 24	0(63) 15
Chocolate	49(136) 24	52(75)	52(111)	76(124)	80(117)	92(124)	83(121)
Sweets	24(67)	6(57)	22(64)	12(47)	8(47)	36(69)	50(118)
Potatoes and potato products:							
Crisps, corn snacks, etc	56(96)	48(72)	50(82)	83(105)	75(93)	56(81)	103(104)
Chips	594(707)	700(744)	647(731)	473(503)	324(476)	412(537)	633(722)
Potatoes	407(479)	498(528)	460(500)	420(479)	458(494)	466(504)	448(510)

Table 54 (Cont)

Food	One parent families			Two parent families			
	One child	Two or more children	All one parent families	One child	Two children	Three children	Four or more children
Vegetables:							
Carrots	20(50) 17	40(43)	26(45)	29(55)	24(48)	0(59) 23	0(72) 15
Tomatoes	0(123) 15	0(162) 15	0(143) 35	0(112) 75	0(107) 64	18(49)	0(124) 12
Baked beans	0(268) 15	155(232)	110(179)	68(151)	0(233) 79	108(164)	92(155)
Peas	85(96)	54(81)	80(92)	55(88)	66(97)	78(104)	56(73)
Salad vegetables	0(82) 18	7(35)	0(73) 37	0(57) 66	0(76) 71	0(51) 24	0(57) 10
Other vegetables	106(142)	135(179)	130(162)	187(224)	172(216)	184(201)	238(259)
Fruit:							
Citrus fruit	0(208) 15	0(215) 14	0(212) 32	0(255) 69	0(211) 67	0(206) 22	0(295) 14
Apples and pears	0(366) 14	0(217) 16	0(287) 30	94(166)	94(171)	120(206)	68(164)
Other fresh fruit	0(182) 10	0(164) 7	0(175) 17	0(183) 29	0(171) 44	0(176) 18	0(87) 8
Other fruit	0(97) 12	0(58) 13	0(9) 27	0(126) 24	0(108) 58	0(108) 16	0(132) 14

Family composition

207

Table 54 (Cont)

Food	Family composition						
	One parent families			Two parent families			
	One child	Two or more children	All one parent families	One child	Two children	Three children	Four or more children
Nuts:							
Nuts	0(0) 0	0(21) 5	0(37) 6	0(39) 13	0(27) 14	0(28) 5	0(39) 6
Peanut butter	0(169) 1	0(73) 2	0(47) 6	0(34) 14	0(22) 15	0(69) 5	0(12) 2
Beverages:							
Fruit juices	0(608) 13	10(149) 13	0(426) 31	0(416) 65	0(337) 60	0(351) 24	0(191) 7
Tea	345(1,309)	799(1,216)	710(1,362)	1,070(1,427)	1,002(1,396)	1,476(1,425)	1,192(1,618)
Coffee	9(45)	6(58)	9(57)	3(27)	6(69)	4(30)	3(52)
Cocoa, drinking chocolate, etc	0(20) 9	0(43) 7	0(30) 16	0(30) 30	0(27) 29	0(25) 15	0(17) 7
Horlicks, Ovaltine	0(199) 16	0(14) 7	0(21) 16	0(24) 28	0(31) 23	0(18) 3	0(24) 9
Milk shakes	0(0) 0	0(0) 0	0(0) 0	0(300) 1	0(0) 0	0(0) 0	0(0) 0
Colas	0(601) 14	0(741) 13	0(644) 31	0(615) 72	0(601) 67	0(319) 19	0(658) 12
Fizzy drinks	446(800)	388(494)	330(638)	250(491)	244(473)	330(416)	296(474)
Other soft drinks	0(199) 16	0(180) 14	0(178) 32	0(246) 55	0(248) 63	0(234) 24	0(266) 15

Table 54 (Cont)

Food	Family composition						
	One parent families			Two parent families			
	One child	Two or more children	All one parent families	One child	Two children	Three children	Four or more children
Alcoholic drinks:							
Beers and lagers	0(394) 2	0(159) 2	0(250) 4	0(467) 15	0(310) 11	0(152) 4	0(0) 0
Wines	0(138) 3	9(306) 8	0(240) 8	0(315) 12	0(159) 8	0(232) 4	0(0) 0
Spirits	0(0) 0	0(0) 0	0(117) 2	0(66) 2	0(23) 5	0(0) 0	0(0) 0
Other foods:							
Pickles and sauces	13(43) 14	10(44) 16	10(44) 31	12(39) 77	10(37) 5	24(48) 13	10(36) 13
Soups	0(405)	0(445)	0(422)	0(346)	120(187)	234(297)	0(463)
Number of children	38	33	75	159	142	52	35

Table 55: *Foods consumed by girls aged 14/15 years (g/head/week)*

Food	Employment and benefits (benefits are also received by one-parent families)				
	Father unemployed	Father in employment	Family Income Supplement (FIS)	Supplementary Benefit (SB)	Neither FIS or SB
Number of children	70	312	10	71	368
Cereals:					
White bread	467(537)	432(466)	489(566)	433(491)	432(476)
Brown bread	0(147) 12	0(166) 52	0(0) 0	0(177) 9	0(158) 62
Wholemeal bread	0(256) 12	0(217) 77	0(95) 2	0(259) 9	0(212) 90
Other bread	0(157) 22	0(141) 91	0(0) 0	0(180) 22	0(137) 108
Total bread	(653)	(578)	(591)	(604)	(591)
Bran products	0(0) 0	0(117) 17	0(0) 0	0(0) 0	0(118) 19
Buns and pastries	0(139) 33	37(68)	25(52)	38(70)	30(68)
Cakes	110(156)	118(166)	168(190)	128(161)	112(162)
Biscuits	137(172)	116(145)	111(139)	128(162)	118(148)
Breakfast cereals	46(112)	83(124)	73(103)	88(144)	71(119)
Puddings, etc	224(270)	222(262)	132(249)	204(243)	222(271)
Icecream	0(122) 18	0(93) 102	30(56)	0(116) 17	0(98) 124
Rice	0(255) 16	0(264) 80	0(559) 3	0(252) 27	0(252) 83
Pasta	0(234) 23	0(219) 119	0(187) 4	0(204) 20	0(226) 144

Table 55 (Cont)

Food	Employment and benefits (benefits are also received by one-parent families)				
	Father unemployed	Father in employment	Family Income Supplement (FIS)	Supplementary Benefit (SB)	Neither FIS or SB
Milk and milk products:					
Cows milk, whole	954(1,120)	1,221(1,334)	914(1,171)	945(1,140)	1,181(1,329)
Skimmed, semi skimmed milk	0(481) 5	0(729) 7	0(260) 1	0(541) 6	0(670) 9
Other milk	0(31) 6	0(102) 34	0(0) 0	0(41) 11	0(85) 39
Yogurt	0(214) 19	0(274) 86	0(423) 3	0(196) 16	0(273) 104
Cream	0(34) 16	0(44) 85	0(32) 5	0(41) 16	0(44) 94
Cottage cheese	0(43) 2	0(54) 11	0(0) 0	0(0) 0	0(77) 14
Cheese	60(109)	76(107)	90(128)	33(84)	76(109)
Eggs, egg dishes	146(167)	92(108)	108(128)	104(153)	92(111)
Fats and oils:					
Butter	15(41)	29(47)	49(64)	10(37)	28(46)
Margarine	28(41)	8(34)	17(23)	22(37)	10(36)
Low fat spread	0(0) 0	0(25) 6	0(0) 0	0(0) 0	0(41) 9
Vegetable oils	0(14) 4	0(19) 10	0(0) 0	0(12) 7	0(17) 11
Other fats and oils	0(13) 1	0(46) 22	0(14) 1	0(0) 0	0(43) 26

Table 55 (Cont)

Food	Employment and benefits (benefits are also received by one-parent families)				
	Father unemployed	Father in employment	Family Income Supplement (FIS)	Supplementary Benefit (SB)	Neither FIS or SB
Carcase meats:					
Bacon and ham	32(47)	48(61)	37(52)	38(45)	42(61)
Beef and veal	0(121) 31	48(86)	0(45) 2	0(177) 29	43(82)
Mutton and lamb	0(200) 25	0(124) 94	0(112) 5	0(226) 21	0(121) 116
Pork	0(107) 32	0(122) 140	0(129) 3	0(118) 26	0(119) 173
Other meat:					
Chicken fried in breadcrumbs	0(0) 0	0(99) 7	0(0) 0	0(148) 1	0(106) 8
Poultry and game	43(73)	76(110)	0(137) 4	34(82)	74(110)
Liver	0(88) 18	0(83) 68	0(0) 0	0(96) 15	0(82) 79
Kidney	0(20) 3	0(0) 0	0(0) 0	0(0) 0	0(19) 3
Other offals	0(84) 1	0(68) 11	0(0) 0	0(53) 2	0(74) 12
Sausages	80(105)	46(77)	34(117)	66(96)	48(122)
Burgers	0(42) 32	0(104) 111	0(99) 3	36(62)	0(102) 149
Other meat products	320(389)	306(355)	428(448)	351(397)	306(354)

Table 55 (Cont)

Food	Employment and benefits (benefits are also received by one-parent families)				
	Father unemployed	Father in employment	Family Income Supplement (FIS)	Supplementary Benefit (SB)	Neither FIS or SB
Fish and fish products:					
Fish in batter or breadcrumbs	0(151)	0(138)	0(171)	0(139)	0(133)
	24	91	2	26	144
Fish fingers	0(90)	0(94)	0(126)	0(113)	0(96)
	16	85	4	21	98
Shellfish	0(0)	0(34)	0(0)	0(0)	0(38)
	0	9	0	0	11
Other fish	0(58)	0(87)	0(196)	0(67)	0(82)
	29	100	3	29	115
Sugar, sweets:					
Sugar	130(131)	80(106)	65(96)	119(145)	81(106)
Syrup and preserves	0(52)	0(43)	0(26)	0(33)	0(49)
	28	143	3	26	170
Chocolate	68(86)	84(125)	58(73)	52(108)	80(122)
Sweets	37(69)	12(56)	30(91)	40(75)	13(52)
Potatoes and potato products:					
Crisps, corn snacks, etc	75(90)	78(96)	105(89)	75(94)	77(96)
Chips	530(612)	392(539)	846(795)	680(770)	400(502)
Potatoes	407(481)	432(492)	426(453)	492(495)	426(494)

Table 55 (Cont)

Food	Employment and benefits (benefits are also received by one-parent families)				
	Father unemployed	Father in employment	Family Income Supplement (FIS)	Supplementary Benefit (SB)	Neither FIS or SB
Vegetables:					
Carrots	10(41)	24(47)	0(93) 5	0(83) 33	24(48)
Tomatoes	0(105) 29	0(104) 154	0(131) 4	0(131) 32	0(110) 180
Baked beans	110(174)	45(125)	191(257)	130(188)	50(131)
Peas	66(96)	60(86)	55(112)	77(98)	62(90)
Salad vegetables	0(63) 23	0(64) 151	0(51) 5	0(47) 19	0(68) 182
Other vegetables	170(200)	187(214)	90(159)	170(186)	177(218)
Fruit:					
Citrus fruit	0(246) 22	0(224) 143	0(154) 4	0(232) 24	0(234) 172
Apples and pears	64(140)	102(169)	118(149)	0(273) 30	98(174)
Other fresh fruit	0(141) 18	0(176) 81	0(170) 2	0(169) 18	0(170) 97
Other fruit	0(134) 25	0(109) 125	0(102) 5	0(118) 24	0(112) 146
Nuts:					
Nuts	0(27) 8	0(38) 27	0(70) 2	0(25) 7	0(34) 35
Peanut butter	0(35) 3	0(34) 33	0(94) 2	0(26) 5	0(35) 33

Table 55 (Cont)

Food	Employment and benefits (benefits are also received by one-parent families)				
	Father unemployed	Father in employment	Family Income Supplement (FIS)	Supplementary Benefit (SB)	Neither FIS or SB
Beverages:					
Fruit juices	0(410)	0(369)	0(396)	0(361)	0(377)
	17	139	4	19	163
Tea	1,405(1,787)	1,002(1,341)	354(1,028)	1,267(1,632)	896(1,080)
Coffee	4(45)	5(48)	0(84)	6(64)	4(43)
			5		
Cocoa, drinking chocolate, etc.	0(21)	0(27)	0(40)	0(28)	0(26)
	15	67	3	17	76
Horlicks, Ovaltine	0(29)	0(24)	0(15)	0(22)	0(26)
	17	50	5	15	63
Milk shakes	0(0)	0(300)	0(0)	0(0)	0(300)
	0	1	0	0	1
Colas	0(358)	0(680)	0(384)	0(445)	0(642)
	28	135	3	26	169
Fizzy drinks	222(448)	280(519)	384(516)	319(580)	260(487)
Other soft drinks	0(268)	0(244)	0(131)	0(182)	0(252)
	33	121	3	32	152
Alcoholic drinks:					
Beers and lagers	0(473)	0(367)	0(0)	0(333)	0(357)
	4	26	0	4	31
Wines	0(409)	0(216)	0(509)	0(0)	0(237)
	1	25	2	0	30
Spirits	0(0)	0(52)	0(0)	0(0)	0(51)
	0	8	0	0	8

Table 55 (Cont)

Food	Employment and benefits (benefits are also received by one-parent families)				
	Father unemployed	Father in employment	Family Income Supplement (FIS)	Supplementary Benefit (SB)	Neither FIS or SB
Other foods:					
Pickles and sauces	10(32)	13(42)	35(37)	8(42)	13(40)
Soups	150(216)	52(185)	198(247)	0(418)	78(194)
				27	
Number of children	70	312	10	71	368

Table 56: *Food consumed by girls aged 14/15 years (g/head/week)*

Food	Type of lunch						
	Paid school meal	Free school meal	Paid school meal most days	Free school meal most days	Home	Packed lunch	Cafe
Number of children	72	38	56	19	101	121	54
Cereals:							
White bread	347(416)	452(515)	363(406)	445(526)	463(488)	143(546)	403(463)
Brown bread	0(78)	0(124)	0(92)	0(164)	0(137)	0(214)	0(163)
	4	3	11	1	13	28	10
Wholemeal bread	0(210)	0(12)	0(153)	0(0)	0(177)	0(291)	0(89)
	12	6	15	0	17	42	6
Other bread	0(224)	0(192)	0(99)	0(90)	0(225)	0(98)	0(63)
	24	8	18	6	21	35	17
Total bread	(531)	(588)	(497)	(566)	(584)	(738)	(524)
Bran products	0(56)	0(0)	0(0)	0(7)	0(163)	0(142)	0(95)
	2	0	0	1	2	11	2
Buns and pastries	49(70)	52(79)	46(87)	0(146)	2(52)	42(64)	0(174)
			24	9			25
Cakes	146(227)	161(199)	144(199)	172(164)	80(124)	104(150)	99(114)
Biscuits	100(149)	135(180)	119(140)	88(135)	102(129)	149(178)	85(137)
Breakfast cereals	41(98)	88(142)	110(137)	116(135)	41(95)	111(148)	63(120)
Puddings, etc	196(230)	231(283)	194(231)	286(310)	268(299)	208(280)	210(240)
Icecream	0(104)	0(135)	0(91)	0(35)	0(78)	0(120)	0(84)
	27	16	21	3	31	34	12
Rice	0(214)	0(285)	0(301)	0(282)	0(319)	0(246)	0(219)
	20	13	14	6	16	38	10
Pasta	0(270)	0(196)	0(220)	0(84)	0(220)	0(221)	0(196)
	28	16	24	2	42	35	21

Table 56 (Cont)

Food	Type of lunch						
	Paid school meal	Free school meal	Paid school meal most days	Free school meal most days	Home	Packed lunch	Cafe
Milk and milk products:							
Cows milk, whole	1,266(1,329)	914(1,324)	1,354(1,033)	1,028(1,528)	1,198(1,125)	1,175(1,310)	1,240(1,273)
Skimmed, semi skimmed milk	0(831)	0(583)	0(687)	0(1,000)	0(212)	0(604)	0(0)
	2	3	2	1	2	6	0
Other milk	0(37)	0(50)	0(20)	0(27)	0(111)	0(140)	0(70)
	10	3	2	4	10	15	5
Yogurt	0(183)	0(290)	0(247)	0(313)	0(249)	0(315)	0(243)
	15	11	17	2	26	40	11
Cream	0(45)	0(23)	0(24)	0(38)	0(45)	0(36)	0(131)
	20	11	16	6	26	29	8
Cottage cheese	0(33)	0(2)	0(0)	0(0)	0(0)	0(92)	0(0)
	4	1	0	0	0	10	
Cheese	75(132)	44(100)	77(123)	20(76)	58(87)	94(117)	58(85)
Eggs, egg dishes	75(113)	95(123)	114(133)	79(123)	113(128)	96(107)	68(111)
Fats and oils:							
Butter	33(41)	16(38)	35(46)	5(21)	16(37)	37(61)	30(45)
Margarine	6(23)	12(34)	9(27)	25(43)	16(35)	23(53)	5(22)
Low fat spread	0(17)	0(0)	0(0)	0(0)	0(41)	0(52)	0(0)
	1	0	0	0	2	5	0
Vegetable oils	0(0)	0(20)	0(13)	0(0)	0(16)	0(19)	0(18)
	0	3	4	0	1	5	2
Other fats and oils	0(33)	0(14)	0(10)	0(0)	0(52)	0(61)	0(0)
	9	1	4	0	6	8	0

Table 56 (Cont)

Food	Type of lunch						
	Paid school meal	Free school meal	Paid school meal most days	Free school meal most days	Home	Packed lunch	Cafe
Carcase meats:							
Bacon and ham	33(50)	30(42)	50(67)	0(41) 6	32(57)	53(71)	40(59)
Beef and veal	0(134) 30	0(151) 15	70(111)	0(293) 6	70(87)	40(81)	0(125) 24
Mutton and lamb	0(117) 23	0(129) 15	0(148) 15	0(90) 5	0(178) 24	0(127) 46	0(138) 12
Pork	16(70)	0(83) 14	0(112) 24	0(126) 7	41(64)	0(128) 46	0(88) 15
Other meat:							
Chicken fried in breadcrumbs	0(107) 3	0(0) 0	0(96) 2	0(10) 1	0(94) 1	0(114) 2	0(0) 0
Poultry and game	52(84)	0(143) 17	80(112)	0(120) 7	65(98)	92(133)	88(118)
Liver	0(102) 13	0(73) 7	0(89) 6	0(100) 1	0(80) 25	0(84) 33	0(71) 9
Kidney	0(0) 0	0(0) 0	0(16) 2	0(0) 0	0(27) 2	0(0) 0	0(0) 0
Other offals	0(59) 2	0(0) 0	0(68) 2	0(0) 0	0(95) 5	0(51) 4	0(0) 0
Sausages	68(95)	34(56)	46(78)	114(121)	53(87)	54(81)	0(109) 25
Burgers	0(112) 34	41(66)	20(57)	70(88)	0(86) 30	0(97) 44	0(97) 17
Other meat products	316(365)	428(451)	346(361)	441(427)	278(341)	304(329)	308(383)

Table 56 (Cont)

Food	Type of lunch						
	Paid school meal	Free school meal	Paid school meal most days	Free school meal most days	Home	Packed lunch	Cafe
Fish and fish products:							
Fish in batter or breadcrumbs	0(121)	0(152)	0(125)	0(129)	0(139)	0(139)	0(157)
	22	13	14	9	36	31	15
Fish fingers	0(138)	0(99)	0(94)	0(136)	0(105)	0(80)	0(89)
	24	14	14	7	30	21	13
Shellfish	0(11)	0(0)	0(30)	0(0)	0(51)	0(42)	0(0)
	1	0	2	0	3	4	0
Other fish	0(55)	0(77)	0(70)	14(21)	0(88)	0(90)	0(78)
	13	12	13	14	32	48	18
Sugar, sweets:							
Sugar	78(102)	75(125)	93(104)	149(183)	92(120)	67(102)	95(109)
Syrup and preserves	0(51)	0(29)	0(46)	0(11)	0(46)	0(52)	0(39)
	35	12	26	6	46	54	20
Chocolate	55(118)	48(124)	99(130)	106(147)	92(124)	67(92)	116(152)
Sweets	8(52)	40(90)	17(46)	60(99)	19(69)	8(40)	25(55)
Potatoes and potato products:							
Crisps, corn snacks, etc	50(84)	95(95)	80(97)	35(64)	69(95)	79(100)	100(116)
Chips	666(673)	993(955)	562(609)	770(762)	362(432)	225(314)	606(728)
Potatoes	492(554)	425(468)	404(433)	428(517)	422(497)	425(499)	425(441)

Table 56 (Cont)

Food	Type of lunch						
	Paid school meal	Free school meal	Paid school meal most days	Free school meal most days	Home	Packed lunch	Cafe
Vegetables:							
Carrots	29(49)	26(44)	34(50)	0(90) 8	0(102) 42	30(53)	0(69) 24
Tomatoes	15(56)	0(146) 13	0(130) 26	22(67)	0(127) 39	15(60)	0(74) 25
Baked beans	30(190)	132(210)	34(129)	130(212)	92(150)	24(94)	75(129)
Peas	66(89)	76(98)	56(66)	119(122)	82(110)	56(82)	76(90)
Salad vegetables	10(40)	0(62) 9	3(26)	0(42) 4	0(59) 39	8(43)	0(41) 25
Other vegetables	198(258)	158(182)	122(159)	164(149)	180(208)	234(253)	132(163)
Fruit:							
Citrus fruit	0(252) 33	0(143) 12	0(216) 24	0(168) 8	0(206) 41	45(150)	0(200) 21
Apples and pears	90(132)	0(209) 18	0(222) 27	0(263) 8	0(351) 50	168(257)	11(116)
Other fresh fruit	0(170) 17	0(150) 5	0(138) 16	0(109) 5	0(177) 27	0(188) 32	0(177) 14
Other fruit	0(116) 27	0(80) 10	0(83) 22	0(96) 7	0(50) 41	0(110) 46	0(92) 22
Nuts:							
Nuts	0(22) 3	0(41) 5	0(31) 7	0(20) 1	0(38) 12	0(31) 12	0(36) 3
Peanut butter	0(19) 2	0(70) 3	0(32) 6	0(12) 3	0(48) 10	0(35) 12	0(13) 3

Table 56 (Cont)

Food	Type of lunch						
	Paid school meal	Free school meal	Paid school meal most days	Free school meal most days	Home	Packed lunch	Cafe
Beverages:							
Fruit juices	0(367) / 29	0(228) / 11	0(440) / 26	0(308) / 5	0(312) / 31	0(447) / 58	0(321) / 24
Tea	400(1,070)	1,002(1,220)	1,002(1,135)	1,150(1,368)	1,426(1,757)	1,349(1,575)	528(1,261)
Coffee	4(76)	4(28)	4(18)	13(56)	6(44)	4(56)	7(27)
Cocoa, drinking chocolate, etc	0(23) / 18	0(38) / 11	0(31) / 16	0(16) / 3	0(31) / 16	0(28) / 24	0(28) / 8
Horlicks, Ovaltine	0(30) / 16	0(29) / 13	0(20) / 14	0(19) / 2	0(20) / 10	0(23) / 19	0(29) / 7
Milk shakes	0(0) / 0	0(0) / 0	0(0) / 0	0(0) / 0	0(0) / 0	0(300) / 1	0(0) / 0
Colas	0(575) / 28	0(442) / 13	30(300) / 13	0(423) / 6	0(715) / 45	0(578) / 47	100(360)
Fizzy drinks	302(455)	384(648)	426(597)	330(683)	200(370)	180(446)	507(669)
Other soft drinks	0(230) / 33	0(147) / 16	0(390) / 25	44(88)	0(269) / 29	0(231) / 52	0(158) / 20
Alcoholic drinks:							
Beers and lagers	0(320) / 9	0(416) / 3	0(723) / 6	0(9) / 1	0(313) / 4	0(173) / 9	0(302) / 2
Wines	0(105) / 3	0(9) / 1	0(116) / 7	0(0) / 0	0(247) / 8	0(187) / 10	0(356) / 3
Spirits	0(30) / 2	0(0) / 0	0(4) / 1	0(0) / 0	0(98) / 2	0(66) / 2	0(35) / 2

Table 56 (Cont)

Food	Type of lunch						
	Paid school meal	Free school meal	Paid school meal most days	Free school meal most days	Home	Packed lunch	Cafe
Other foods:							
Pickles and sauces	12(58)	17(40)	10(32)	10(33)	0(58) 49	17(46)	16(35)
Soups	0(376) 32	0(347) 13	0(327) 24	56(205)	222(303)	0(349) 55	78(161)
Number of children	72	38	56	19	101	121	54

Table 57: *Foods consumed by girls aged 14/15 years (g/head/week)*

Food	Type of school meal (excludes those not taking a school meal)		
	Cafeteria	Fixed price	Other
Number of children	162	22	0
Cereals:			
White bread	373(440)	520(475)	(*)
Brown bread	0(92)	0(187)	(*)
	19	1	
Wholemeal bread	0(164)	0(0)	(*)
	33	0	
Other bread	0(142)	0(329)	(*)
	48	7	
Total bread	(527)	(603)	(*)
Bran products	0(117)	0(0)	(*)
	2	0	
Buns and pastries	50(76)	64(86)	(*)
Cakes	144(208)	216(194)	(*)
Biscuits	118(151)	78(118)	(*)
Breakfast cereals	80(130)	36(93)	(*)
Puddings, etc	196(234)	341(355)	(*)
Icecream	0(112)	0(56)	(*)
	58	10	
Rice	0(263)	0(254)	(*)
	45	7	
Pasta	0(234)	0(201)	(*)
	62	8	
Milk and milk products:			
Cows milk, whole	1,068(1,343)	861(1,043)	(*)
Skimmed, semi skimmed milk	0(426)	0(1,178)	(*)
	5	3	
Other milk	0(40)	0(17)	(*)
	16	4	
Yogurt	0(243)	0(179)	(*)
	42	3	
Cream	0(35)	0(12)	(*)
	48	4	
Cottage cheese	0(43)	0(0)	(*)
	4	0	
Cheese	75(124)	30(67)	(*)
Eggs, egg dishes	93(124)	59(106)	(*)
Fats and oils:			
Butter	26(42)	10(23)	(*)
Margarine	9(27)	31(38)	(*)
Low fat spread	0(19)	0(0)	(*)
	2	0	
Vegetable oils	0(14)	0(12)	(*)
	8	1	
Other fats and oils	0(24)	0(35)	(*)
	12	1	

224

Table 57 (Cont)

Food	Type of school meal (excludes those not taking a school meal)		
	Cafeteria	Fixed price	Other
Carcase meats:			
Bacon and ham	36(53)	16(25)	(*)
Beef and veal	0(172)	27(83)	(*)
	73		
Mutton and lamb	0(128)	0(113)	(*)
	52	7	
Pork	0(116)	0(154)	(*)
	73	8	
Other meat:			
Chicken fried in breadcrumbs	0(121)	0(0)	(*)
	5	0	
Poultry and game	48(79)	118(131)	(*)
Liver	0(94)	0(54)	(*)
	26	2	
Kidney	0(16)	0(0)	(*)
	2	0	
Other offals	0(70)	0(48)	(*)
	3	1	
Sausages	50(80)	114(117)	(*)
Burgers	20(57)	68(79)	(*)
Other meat products	334(382)	444(425)	(*)
Fish and fish products:			
Fish in batter or breadcrumbs	0(132)	0(117)	(*)
	162	8	
Fish fingers	0(100)	0(166)	(*)
	53	6	
Shellfish	0(18)	0(0)	(*)
	2	0	
Other fish	0(64)	0(48)	(*)
	41	7	
Sugar, sweets:			
Sugar	87(117)	85(105)	(*)
Syrup and preserves	0(44)	0(42)	(*)
	72	7	
Chocolate	68(124)	68(142)	(*)
Sweets	24(66)	10(36)	(*)
Potatoes and potato products:			
Crisps, corn snacks, etc	62(88)	80(93)	(*)
Chips	706(730)	659(647)	(*)
Potatoes	448(492)	424(518)	(*)
Vegetables:			
Carrots	26(48)	54(44)	(*)
Tomatoes	0(118)	0(109)	(*)
	80	10	
Baked beans	90(182)	54(145)	(*)
Peas	66(85)	112(99)	(*)
Salad vegetables	0(65)	0(51)	(*)
	73	7	
Other vegetables	160(204)	164(185)	(*)

225

Table 57 (Cont)

Food	Type of school meal (excludes those not taking a school meal)		
	Cafeteria	Fixed price	Other
Fruit:			
Citrus fruit	0(233)	0(113)	(*)
	71	6	
Apples and pears	0(237)	91(114)	(*)
	79		
Other fresh fruit	0(154)	0(123)	(*)
	35	7	
Other fruit	0(97)	0(95)	(*)
	61	5	
Nuts:			
Nuts	0(34)	0(8)	(*)
	15	2	
Peanut butter	0(34)	0(38)	(*)
	13	1	
Beverages:			
Fruit juices	0(393)	0(140)	(*)
	64	7	
Tea	674(1,154)	470(1,153)	(*)
Coffee	4(52)	0(24)	(*)
		10	
Cocoa, drinking chocolate, etc	0(29)	0(7)	(*)
	46	2	
Horlicks, Ovaltine	0(24)	0(33)	(*)
	35	10	
Milk shakes	0(0)	0(0)	(*)
	0	0	
Colas	0(536)	0(604)	(*)
	67	8	
Fizzy drinks	354(547)	396(660)	(*)
Other soft drinks	0(208)	0(676)	(*)
	76	8	
Alcoholic drinks:			
Beers and lagers	0(417)	0(0)	(*)
	19	0	
Wines	0(135)	0(0)	(*)
	10	0	
Spirits	0(19)	0(0)	(*)
	4	0	
Other foods:			
Pickles and sauces	13(45)	10(38)	(*)
Soups	0(377)	78(148)	(*)
	16		
Number of children	162	22	0

List of Figures

Figure 6.1
DAILY INTAKE OF ENERGY (MJ)

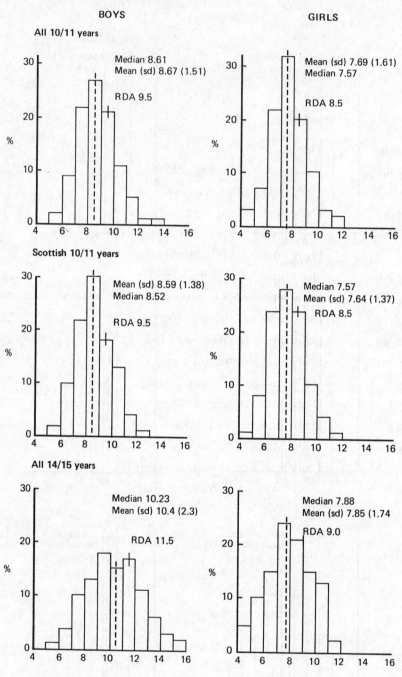

BOYS   GIRLS

All 10/11 years

Median 8.61
Mean (sd) 8.67 (1.51)
RDA 9.5

Mean (sd) 7.69 (1.61)
Median 7.57
RDA 8.5

Scottish 10/11 years

Mean (sd) 8.59 (1.38)
Median 8.52
RDA 9.5

Median 7.57
Mean (sd) 7.64 (1.37)
RDA 8.5

All 14/15 years

Median 10.23
Mean (sd) 10.4 (2.3)
RDA 11.5

Median 7.88
Mean (sd) 7.85 (1.74
RDA 9.0

228

Figure 6.2
DAILY INTAKE OF PROTEIN (g)

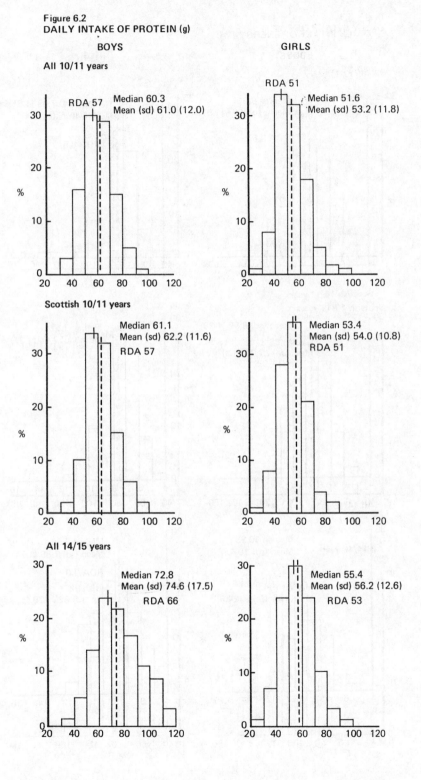

BOYS

GIRLS

All 10/11 years

RDA 57 Median 60.3 Mean (sd) 61.0 (12.0)

RDA 51 Median 51.6 Mean (sd) 53.2 (11.8)

Scottish 10/11 years

Median 61.1 Mean (sd) 62.2 (11.6) RDA 57

Median 53.4 Mean (sd) 54.0 (10.8) RDA 51

All 14/15 years

Median 72.8 Mean (sd) 74.6 (17.5) RDA 66

Median 55.4 Mean (sd) 56.2 (12.6) RDA 53

Figure 6.3
DAILY INTAKE OF FAT (g)

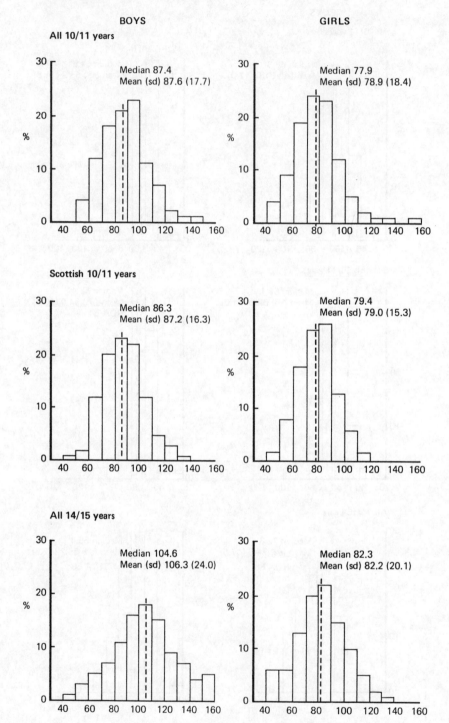

BOYS

GIRLS

All 10/11 years

Median 87.4
Mean (sd) 87.6 (17.7)

Median 77.9
Mean (sd) 78.9 (18.4)

Scottish 10/11 years

Median 86.3
Mean (sd) 87.2 (16.3)

Median 79.4
Mean (sd) 79.0 (15.3)

All 14/15 years

Median 104.6
Mean (sd) 106.3 (24.0)

Median 82.3
Mean (sd) 82.2 (20.1)

Figure 6.4
DAILY INTAKE OF FAT AS PERCENTAGE OF ENERGY INTAKE

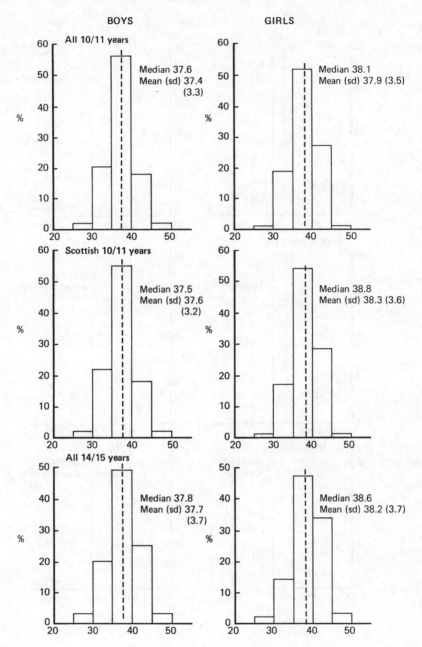

BOYS

All 10/11 years
Median 37.6
Mean (sd) 37.4 (3.3)

Scottish 10/11 years
Median 37.5
Mean (sd) 37.6 (3.2)

All 14/15 years
Median 37.8
Mean (sd) 37.7 (3.7)

GIRLS

Median 38.1
Mean (sd) 37.9 (3.5)

Median 38.8
Mean (sd) 38.3 (3.6)

Median 38.6
Mean (sd) 38.2 (3.7)

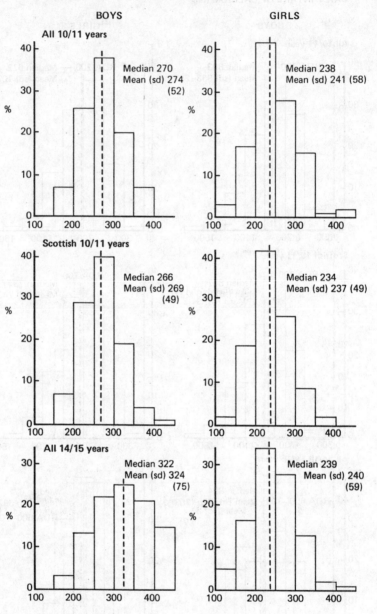

Figure 6.5
DAILY INTAKE OF CARBOHYDRATE (g)

BOYS

GIRLS

All 10/11 years

Median 270
Mean (sd) 274
(52)

Median 238
Mean (sd) 241 (58)

Scottish 10/11 years

Median 266
Mean (sd) 269
(49)

Median 234
Mean (sd) 237 (49)

All 14/15 years

Median 322
Mean (sd) 324
(75)

Median 239
Mean (sd) 240
(59)

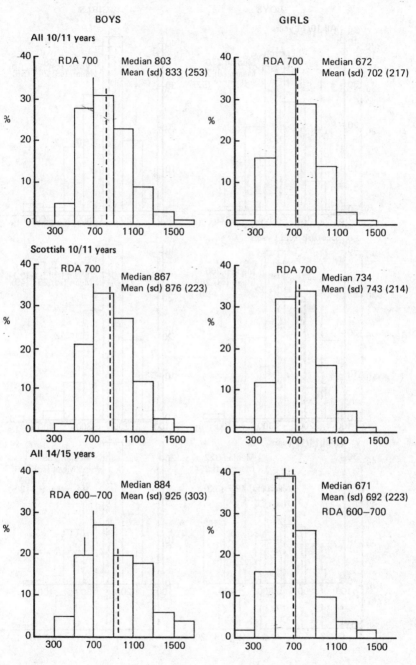

Figure 6.6
DAILY INTAKE OF CALCIUM (mg)

BOYS

GIRLS

All 10/11 years

RDA 700   Median 803
Mean (sd) 833 (253)

RDA 700   Median 672
Mean (sd) 702 (217)

Scottish 10/11 years

RDA 700   Median 867
Mean (sd) 876 (223)

RDA 700   Median 734
Mean (sd) 743 (214)

All 14/15 years

RDA 600–700   Median 884
Mean (sd) 925 (303)

Median 671
Mean (sd) 692 (223)
RDA 600–700

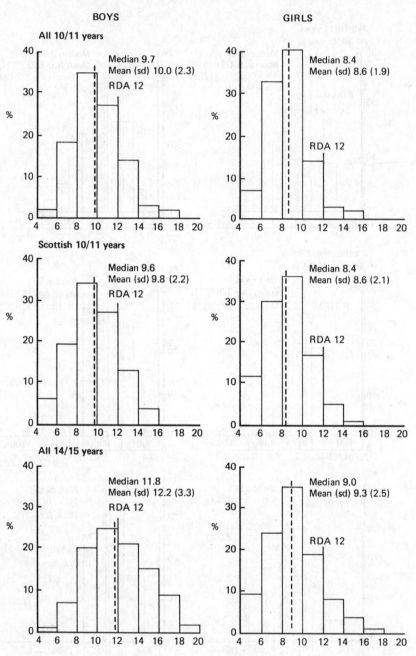

Figure 6.7
DAILY INTAKE OF IRON (mg)

BOYS

GIRLS

All 10/11 years

Median 9.7
Mean (sd) 10.0 (2.3)
RDA 12

Median 8.4
Mean (sd) 8.6 (1.9)
RDA 12

Scottish 10/11 years

Median 9.6
Mean (sd) 9.8 (2.2)
RDA 12

Median 8.4
Mean (sd) 8.6 (2.1)
RDA 12

All 14/15 years

Median 11.8
Mean (sd) 12.2 (3.3)
RDA 12

Median 9.0
Mean (sd) 9.3 (2.5)
RDA 12

234

Figure 6.8
DAILY INTAKE OF THIAMIN (mg)

BOYS

GIRLS

All 10/11 years

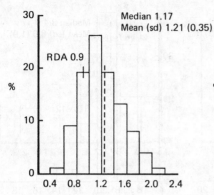

Median 1.17
Mean (sd) 1.21 (0.35)
RDA 0.9

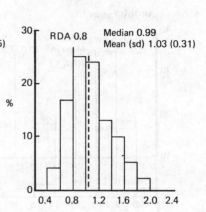

RDA 0.8   Median 0.99
Mean (sd) 1.03 (0.31)

Scottish 10/11 years

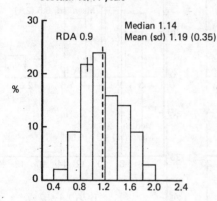

RDA 0.9   Median 1.14
Mean (sd) 1.19 (0.35)

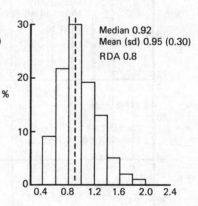

Median 0.92
Mean (sd) 0.95 (0.30)
RDA 0.8

All 14/15 years

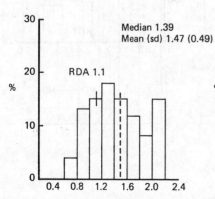

Median 1.39
Mean (sd) 1.47 (0.49)
RDA 1.1

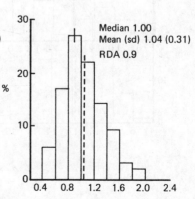

Median 1.00
Mean (sd) 1.04 (0.31)
RDA 0.9

Figure 6.9
DAILY INTAKE OF RIBOFLAVIN (mg)

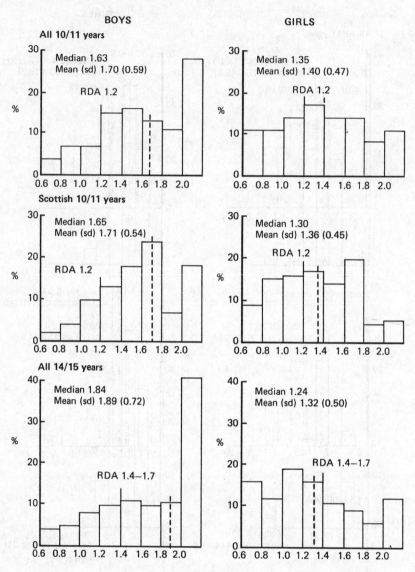

BOYS

All 10/11 years

Median 1.63
Mean (sd) 1.70 (0.59)
RDA 1.2

Scottish 10/11 years

Median 1.65
Mean (sd) 1.71 (0.54)
RDA 1.2

All 14/15 years

Median 1.84
Mean (sd) 1.89 (0.72)
RDA 1.4–1.7

GIRLS

Median 1.35
Mean (sd) 1.40 (0.47)
RDA 1.2

Median 1.30
Mean (sd) 1.36 (0.45)
RDA 1.2

Median 1.24
Mean (sd) 1.32 (0.50)
RDA 1.4–1.7

236

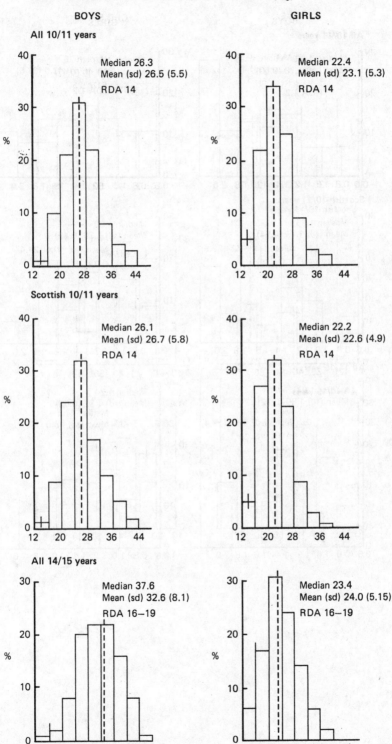

Figure 6.10
DAILY INTAKE OF NICOTINIC ACID EQUIVALENT (mg)

BOYS

GIRLS

All 10/11 years

Median 26.3
Mean (sd) 26.5 (5.5)
RDA 14

Median 22.4
Mean (sd) 23.1 (5.3)
RDA 14

Scottish 10/11 years

Median 26.1
Mean (sd) 26.7 (5.8)
RDA 14

Median 22.2
Mean (sd) 22.6 (4.9)
RDA 14

All 14/15 years

Median 37.6
Mean (sd) 32.6 (8.1)
RDA 16—19

Median 23.4
Mean (sd) 24.0 (5.15)
RDA 16—19

237

Figure 6.11
DAILY INTAKE OF VITAMIN C (mg)

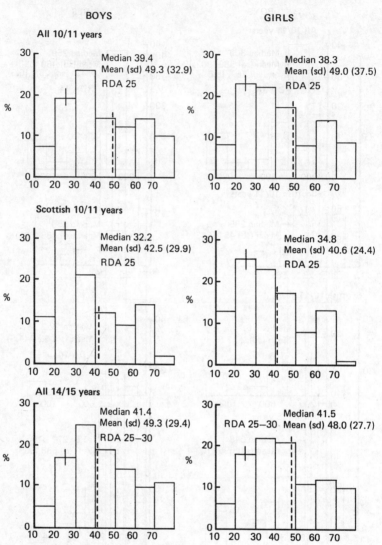

BOYS

GIRLS

All 10/11 years

Median 39.4
Mean (sd) 49.3 (32.9)
RDA 25

Median 38.3
Mean (sd) 49.0 (37.5)
RDA 25

Scottish 10/11 years

Median 32.2
Mean (sd) 42.5 (29.9)
RDA 25

Median 34.8
Mean (sd) 40.6 (24.4)
RDA 25

All 14/15 years

Median 41.4
Mean (sd) 49.3 (29.4)
RDA 25—30

Median 41.5
RDA 25—30 Mean (sd) 48.0 (27.7)

238

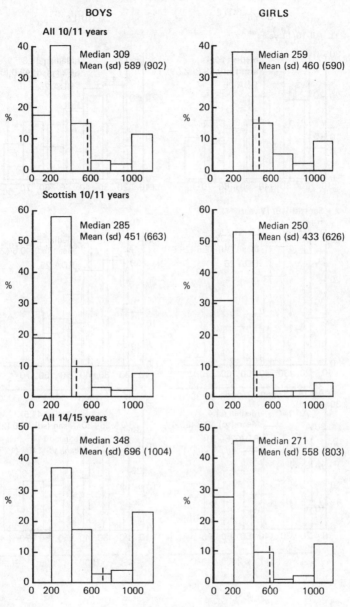

Figure 6.12
DAILY INTAKE OF RETINOL (µg)

BOYS

GIRLS

All 10/11 years

Median 309
Mean (sd) 589 (902)

Median 259
Mean (sd) 460 (590)

Scottish 10/11 years

Median 285
Mean (sd) 451 (663)

Median 250
Mean (sd) 433 (626)

All 14/15 years

Median 348
Mean (sd) 696 (1004)

Median 271
Mean (sd) 558 (803)

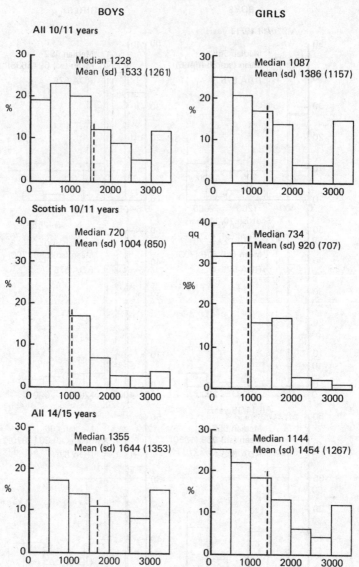

Figure 6.13
DAILY INTAKE OF β–CAROTENE (μg)

BOYS

GIRLS

All 10/11 years

Median 1228
Mean (sd) 1533 (1261)

Median 1087
Mean (sd) 1386 (1157)

Scottish 10/11 years

Median 720
Mean (sd) 1004 (850)

Median 734
Mean (sd) 920 (707)

All 14/15 years

Median 1355
Mean (sd) 1644 (1353)

Median 1144
Mean (sd) 1454 (1267)

Figure 6.14
DAILY INTAKE OF RETINOL EQUIVALENT (µg)

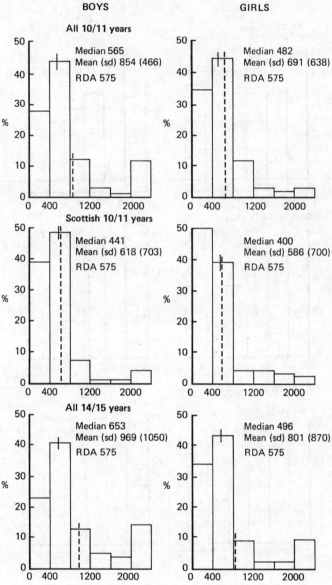

BOYS

GIRLS

All 10/11 years

Median 565
Mean (sd) 854 (466)
RDA 575

Median 482
Mean (sd) 691 (638)
RDA 575

Scottish 10/11 years

Median 441
Mean (sd) 618 (703)
RDA 575

Median 400
Mean (sd) 586 (700)
RDA 575

All 14/15 years

Median 653
Mean (sd) 969 (1050)
RDA 575

Median 496
Mean (sd) 801 (870)
RDA 575

Figure 6.15
DAILY INTAKE OF VITAMIN D (µg)

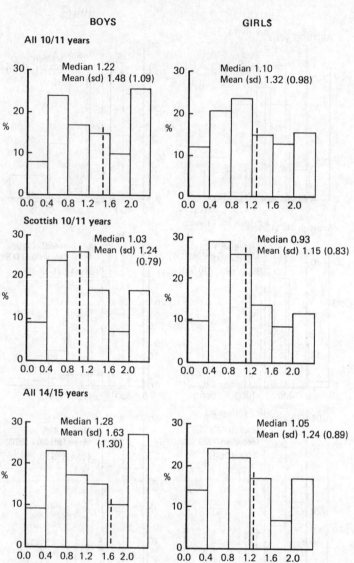

BOYS

GIRLS

All 10/11 years

Median 1.22
Mean (sd) 1.48 (1.09)

Median 1.10
Mean (sd) 1.32 (0.98)

Scottish 10/11 years

Median 1.03
Mean (sd) 1.24
(0.79)

Median 0.93
Mean (sd) 1.15 (0.83)

All 14/15 years

Median 1.28
Mean (sd) 1.63
(1.30)

Median 1.05
Mean (sd) 1.24 (0.89)

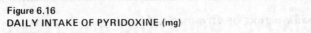

Figure 6.16
DAILY INTAKE OF PYRIDOXINE (mg)

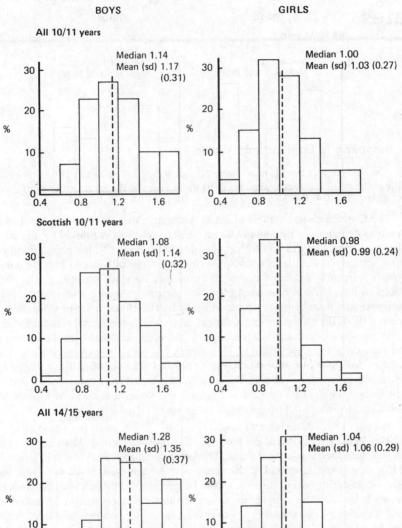

BOYS

GIRLS

All 10/11 years

Median 1.14
Mean (sd) 1.17 (0.31)

Median 1.00
Mean (sd) 1.03 (0.27)

Scottish 10/11 years

Median 1.08
Mean (sd) 1.14 (0.32)

Median 0.98
Mean (sd) 0.99 (0.24)

All 14/15 years

Median 1.28
Mean (sd) 1.35 (0.37)

Median 1.04
Mean (sd) 1.06 (0.29)

Appendix A: Sampling and response rates

1. Sampling in England and Wales

1.1   The sample was based on a multi-stage design to select areas, then schools and finally children in the two groups aged 10 to 14 years at the start of the school year.

1.2   The first stage was a sample of Local Authority Districts from a frame stratified by metropolitan/non-metropolitan counties within standard regions. The aim was to make the selection of districts with probability proportional to the population in the eligible age ranges; but the school address (for allocation to Districts) with the number of pupils were only available in readily accessible form for secondary and middle schools. Although it was possible, at least in England, to secure such information on primary schools from handwritten records held in The Department of Education and Science (DES), the clerical resources required to search the 23,200 files and allocate all primary schools to districts and cumulate the total number of schoolchildren per district could not be made available. However, it was possible to obtain the number of secondary age children for the much smaller number of middle schools so that at least the size of the secondary age population could be counted consistently for all districts. So an initial sample of 64 districts in England and Wales was made with probability proportional to school population aged 11–15 years.

1.3   The geographical area covered by a Local Authority District is usually considerable, especially in rural areas. The survey fieldwork load was very extensive, and if a representative spread of districts was to be achieved, it followed that some degree of clustering within districts would be necessary. Furthermore, to ensure an even sex balance in the sample, single sex secondary schools had to be linked with nearby schools covering the other sex to make a single 'secondary school unit'. Middle school populations of secondary age were linked with the nearest secondary school in the district. Each secondary school unit was then clustered with nearby primary schools so that the primary schools' population was in proportion to the size of the secondary school with which they were clustered. This resulted in clusters containing between 2 and 15 primary schools, some of which proved to cover only children under 9 years of age.

1.4   The survey fieldwork was required at the same time as a major study of schoolchildren's dental health, and the sample design for the two studies was co-ordinated so that DHSS maintained the option of making dental inspections among children in the dietary survey while undertaking the dental survey simply by selecting the same districts for both surveys. However, no school was selected for both surveys since this might have overburdened Local Education Authorities (LEAs), and head teachers, and, in the event, DHSS did not decide to undertake dental inspections of the children in this survey.

244

1.5   Since the dental health survey should have covered all primary school ages, the clusters around the secondary schools include all primary schools in the selected districts, irrespective of the age range covered. Hence, in effect, the primary school population from age 5 to 10 years grouped in this way was used as an approximation for the relative population of children aged 10 years within the clusters.

1.6   Once the schools had been grouped into clusters within the selected districts, one cluster was randomly selected from each sampled district with probability proportional to the size of the secondary age (11 to 15 years) school population in each cluster.

1.7   Having selected the clusters with probability proportional to secondary size, insofar as this represented the eligible ages, a sample of an equal number of children from each selected school cluster would be expected. If, in each cluster, the number of children in the eligible age range were the same proportion within each primary school this would yield an equal sample size in each cluster. However, the proportion in the eligible age range varied between schools and this should theoretically have been allowed for by a fixed sampling fraction, such that some primary school clusters yielded more 10/11 year olds than others. Even in the secondary schools, a predetermined sampling fraction would yield varying sizes of sampling as those schools varied in the proportion of 14/15 year olds they contained.

1.8   However the fieldwork for each child in the survey was so extensive that the interviewers' workload had to be predictable for each selected school. The sifting procedure (described elsewhere) which was required to increase the coverage of social classes IV and V was an important and unavoidable source of variation between schools and any other source of variation would have made interviewer fieldwork assignments unmanageable.

1.9   Hence it was decided that the initial sample size selected in schools should be fixed, and the number of primary schools within each cluster was also fixed at two. In practice, some primary schools were too small to include the required number of children for the survey, so they were grouped within the cluster to form school units expected to contain at least 35 eligible children. It would have been possible to avoid this problem by leaving out small schools but this would have under-represented rural areas which could differ in a number of significant ways. The two primary schools required from each cluster were then selected at random with equal probability in all clusters containing more than two such schools.

1.10   The net result of this process was a sample of children no longer selected with equal probability and to restore the representativeness of the sample it was necessary to weight the sample. This was achieved by counting the number of eligible children on the school roll in each school within the selected areas, and using this later to calculate a weighting factor which restored the balance of the sample to that which would have resulted from equal probability sampling. The calculated weighting factor produced for each school was applied to data from the sampled children in that school at the analysis stage.

1.11   This has been combined with the weighting factor to take account of oversampling of the less advantaged groups (see section 3) and the weight to restore the correct balance of Scotland with England and Wales (see section 2) to produce a composite weight appropriate to each subgroup in the sample. Those composite weights have been applied in all the analyses undertaken for this report. It is essential that anyone using this data set for subsequent analysis should also use those weights if the results are to be characterised as representative of British schoolchildren in the relevant age groups. On the data tapes they have been stored under the variable name GBWEIGHT for the total sample, and SPWEIGHT on the tape which includes only the Scottish primary children.

2. Sampling in Scotland

2.1 *Primary schoolchildren*   The aim of the survey was to interview a representative sample of Scottish children aged 10–11 years defined as the children who had reached the age of 10 at the start of the school year in maintained and grant aided (but not fully independent) schools. Ideally the survey would have included children from all over Scotland but the inordinately high cost of visiting a sample in the offshore islands and the districts north of the Caledonian Canel precluded these areas from the sample. It is estimated from Scottish Education Department (SED) figures provided to OPCS that this unrepresented group account for no more than about 2 per cent of the sampling population. Again, for cost reasons, the sample also excluded schools which SED records showed to contain less than 5 children in the eligible age range and it is estimated that this second unrepresented group account for 1 per cent of the population.

2.2   All Scottish primary schools within the population were grouped in clusters of one or more nearby addresses to make small groups containing at least 70 children of the relevant age group using the most recent SED statistical returns. These clusters were made up to provide reasonably sized geographical areas within which a fieldworker could order all her fieldwork without consuming inordinate resources in travelling between sampled children. The population of schools having been grouped in this way, 52 clusters were then selected with probability proportional to cluster size.

2.3   The listed schools from each selected cluster were visited and sampling frames were constructed from which 40 children of the relevant age were randomly selected, and interviewing then proceeded as in England and Wales.

2.4   The sample of primary children was designed to produce sufficient numbers in Scotland for Scottish estimates to be made. However, when added in with the results for England and Wales to produce estimates for Great Britain, the results from the entire Scottish sample have been weighted down to represent their true proportion within Great Britain.

2.5   Also, as in England and Wales, the children from certain social groups were given a higher probability of selection in order to ensure a large enough subsample for special analysis. However, in the general presentation of results these have been weighted back to their representative proportion within the total sample.

2.6   *The selection of children in secondary schools in Scotland*   Having excluded Secondary schools north of the Caledonian Canal, the remainder were listed within LEAs and 8 were selected from the list with probability proportional to the number of children aged 12–15 years. Within each selected school a random sample of 40 children was taken from the relevant age group and interviewed as in England and Wales. All the resulting interviews have been added in with those from the 14–15 year old children in England and Wales with an appropriate weighting factor to represent them in the correct national ratio.

3. The enhanced subsample of children from less advantaged families

3.1   In planning the survey there was an interest in the nutrition of children from less advantaged homes. In a straightforward random sample of children, those from poorer homes would be a small minority and not large enough to subsample for separate analysis. So to ensure that they were a large enough subsample within this survey, the sample selection procedure was designed to secure more of such children.

3.2   Schools' records from which the sample was selected did not contain uniform background information about childrens' homes and in any event some LEAs would have objected to releasing this information to OPCS. The detailed information required to identify children from less advantaged homes was too complicated to be secured from a postal questionnaire, and therefore a sifting procedure was carried out in the field by the interviewer.

3.3   The parents of a random sample of children were allocated serial numbers and visited at home in order to conduct a short sift interview. If the information gathered at that stage showed that the children were within the special interest group they were automatically eligible for full interview; if not only the cases with odd serial numbers were eligible.

3.4   *Defining the group of interest*   The group of special interest was defined as those children who came from the following backgrounds:

   those with unemployed fathers
   those with fathers disabled or long term sick;
   those from single parent families;
   those from social classes IV and V (where incomes tended to be lower on average).

The unemployed were defined as those currently within the labour market and looking for work. The long term sick were defined as those who saw themselves as sick and out of the labour market, and those who had been off work sick for over a year. Social classes IV and V are the two bottom groups in the Registrar-General's classification of social class. They were defined in terms of the occupation of the head of the family and cover semi-skilled and unskilled, mainly manual work, occupations. Once interviewers had gathered the necessary occupation details they were usually able to establish whether the family fell into social classes IV or V by means of a chart and lists with which they had been issued. Where there was some doubt, interviewers were instructed to phone head office for specialist advice.

3.5   *Representation of the special interest group within the tabulated results*   Within the tables of results in this report the figures for the total sample have been reweighted to restore the less advantaged group to their correct proportion of the total, because the overall results would otherwise be biased towards the situation in the less advantaged homes. However, when the special interest group is analysed separately the larger effective sample enhances the precision of the results for that group.

4. Response rate over the whole sample for Great Britain

4.1   The sample for Scotland was deliberately enhanced in the primary age group to facilitate estimates for Scotland alone. In this report the Scottish figures have been weighted down to provide their due proportion of a Great Britain sample, and their response figures have also been weighted down before being added to those for England and Wales in the response analyses which follow.

4.2 The figures have not however been weighted to compensate for unequal probabilities of selection between school clusters. This was because such weighting was expected to have only a marginal effect on the overall result and could only be justified if very accurate figures for the eligible population were available, which they were not when the whole school refused to co-operate. For the fully responding sample however, this intercluster weighting was undertaken and the 'number of interviews' in the response analysis which follows will not be the same as the figure which features in the tables of substantive results.

4.3 Since the figures in the other tables have been weighted they do not show the actual number of successful records achieved, which were:

	Boys	Girls	Total
Scottish primary age	527	522	1,049
Scottish secondary age	62	59	121
English and Welsh primary age	530	485	1,015
English and Welsh secondary age	567	544	1,111
Total	1,686	1,610	3,296

The weighted response rate achieved was 75.2 per cent and the different sources of nonresponse are given in Table A.

4.4 As with any sample taken from intermediate organisations there was a loss caused by nonresponse from the organisations. In this survey it is estimated that some 4.1 per cent (weighted) was lost from the eligible sample. However that can only be an estimate for it has been based on the assumption that the ineligible children within the refused schools comprised the same proportion as was found in the co-operating schools.

4.5 The refusing schools almost always cited the volume of extra work caused by bodies contacting them for information or access to their children and claimed that they could not accommodate any further requests no matter how worthy the cause.

Table A: *Sample response rates*

	Number	Per cent
Children sampled from school registers	4,597	
Children who would have been sampled if their school had not refused to co-operate	+ 187	
Total potential sample	4,784	
Subtract ineligibles (ill all survey period or moved out of sampled area)	− 50	
Subtract children found to be in the higher social classes I–III non-manual in the sifted sample (see sample design)	−1,436	
Subtract estimated number of refusals and non-contacts which would have been in the higher social classes I–III non-manual and have been ineligible if they had co-operated	− 174	
Total eligible sample	3,124	100.0
Estimated number of children from refusing schools who would have been eligible	129	4.1
Estimated number of non-contacts who would have been eligible if they had been contacted	29	0.9
Estimated number of refusals who would have been eligible if they had co-operated	229	7.3
Number of children who dropped out during the recording period having previously promised to keep 7 day records	179	5.7
Total co-operating sample	2,558	81.9
Number of children who did not keep records accurately enough	138	4.4
Number of children whose recording week included less than 3 schooldays	78	2.3
Number of children for whom satisfactory records were obtained	2,348	75.2

5. Response rate in Scotland

5.1 The number of children aged 10/11 years in Scotland from whom satisfactory records were collected was 1,058. The weighted response rate achieved was 75.2 per cent. The different sources of nonresponse are given in Table B.

5.2 As with any sample taken from intermediate organisations there was a loss caused by nonresponse from the organisations. In this survey it is estimated that some 7.8 per cent (weighted) was lost from the Scottish eligible sample. However that can only be an estimate for it has to be based on the assumption that the ineligible children within the refusing schools comprised the same proportion as found in the co-operating schools.

249

6. Calculation of medians from the weighted data base

6.1 The median consumption in grams per child per week was calculated for the weighted data using the software package SPSS–X. As with any calculation of medians the cases (respondents) must be ranked in order of their value for the variable. The cases are then cumulated until 50 per cent of them have been added up at which point the value of the last case added is the median value. When the cases are weighted it is the *weighted* values of the cases which is cumulated. When the total number of cases is not an even number then the theoretical point at which 50 per cent of cases have been cumulated will fall between two cases (eg if there are 21 cases it will fall between the 10th and 11th cases). The median will then be calculated as a mid point between those two cases, ie by interpolation. The example below shows 20 cases of weighted data which for simplicity have been assigned a weight of 0.5 or 1.0.

Case Number	Case Weight	Cumulative Weight	Value
1	1	1.0	20
2	0.5	1.5	20
3	1	2.5	20
4	1	3.5	22
5	0.5	4.0	23
6	1	5.0	24
7	1	6.0	24
8	1	7.0	24
9	1	8.0	25 — median
10	1	9.0	25
11	1	10.0	27
12	0.5	10.5	28
13	1	11.5	28
14	1	12.5	29
15	0.5	13.0	30
16	0.5	13.5	31
17	0.5	14.0	35
18	0.5	14.5	40
19	0.5	15.0	47
20	1	16.0	48

The data are ranked in order of, say, grams of food in the value column. The cumulative weighted total is 16 so the point at which 50 per cent have been listed is 8, giving a median of 25.

Table B: *Sample response rates in Scotland*

	Number	Per cent
Children sampled from school registers	1,915	
Children who would have been sampled if their school had not refused to co-operate	+ 155	
Total potential sample	2,070	
Subtract ineligibles (ill all survey period or moved out of sampled area)	− 4	
Subtract children found to be in the higher social classes I–III non-manual in the sifted sample (see sample design)	− 590	
Subtract estimated number of refusals and non-contacts which would have been in the higher social classes I–III non-manual and have been ineligible if they had co-operated	− 83	
Total eligible sample	1,393	100.0
Estimated number of children from refusing schools who would have been eligible	108	7.8
Estimated number of non-contacts who would have been eligible if they had been contacted	28	2.0
Estimated number of refusals who would have been eligible if they had co-operated	55	3.9
Number of children who dropped out during the recording period having previously promised to keep 7 day records	78	5.6
Total co-operating sample	1,124	80.7
Number of children who did not keep records accurately enough	66	4.7
Number of children whose recording week included less than 3 schooldays	8	0.6
Number of children for whom satisfactory records were obtained	1,050	75.4

6.2 To enable comparison with other dietary surveys the arithmetic mean is also given (in tables 34 to 57) alongside the median. Some foods were rarely consumed: when more than 50 per cent of the children ate none the median value was therefore zero. For these foods the arithmetic mean weekly consumption of those children who ate the food during the survey week is given in brackets, with the number of children immediately below. No tests of statistical significance have been applied to the differences in patterns of food consumption described in this report. Nevertheless the data have been presented for information in section 9 and some dietary patterns have emerged which are discussed.

Appendix B: The Dietary Survey

1. Selection and training of fieldworkers

1.1 The interviewers were selected from the OPCS panel of fully trained fieldworkers known for their ability to handle complex surveys; their ability to learn large amounts of special information quickly and their availability for fulltime work. The training for this survey began with a postal briefing on the methods and detail of dietary record keeping, followed by a 7 day period of personal diet recording together with a food coding exercise.

1.2 Fieldworkers then attended a 2 day training session during which the principle and practice of probing for detail in dietary records, and more complex food coding, were taught by people experienced in this type of survey. They were also trained to measure the heights and weights of children. Following lectures, practical demonstrations and tests, interviewers were sent away to place a dietary record book with a child who was not a member of their household. This practice fieldwork followed the pattern of work that would be used in the main survey with interviewers making check records and coding their contents for a period of 4 days, including at least one weekend day. The questionnaire, diary and record book are reproduced at the end of this Appendix.

1.3 After 4 days the fieldworkers collected the completed records and brought them to a third full day training session, where training was given in dealing with more complex cases. They were taught how to recognise the limitations of their own nutritional knowledge so that they would know when to telephone a nutritional fieldwork adviser for guidance. Each interviewer had a personal training session with a nutritional fieldworker adviser who discussed with them any problems that had arisen during the 4 day training dietary record.

1.4 The first 3 or 4 records completed in the main survey by each fieldworker were scrutinised in great detail by the nutritionist food coding advisers. Any minor deficiencies were notified to the fieldworkers in writing and any more complex points were explained by telephone. All the allocated food codes were checked on the first few hundred record books to be returned, but thereafter only "leftover" and "split" codes were systematically checked with occasional spot checks on other codes.

2. The Fieldwork Procedure

2.1 With all children, the fieldworker's first step was to explain the nature of the survey to one or both of the parents following up an explanatory letter which has been posted to them. The questionnaire interview then followed, in the course of which the field sift was used to sort out ineligible children.

252

2.2 *The initial interview* The initial questionnaire interview, which collected basic socio-economic data, also included questions about diet and eating patterns. Foods specifically avoided and meals not usually taken were noted to help the fieldworker understand the child's "normal" eating pattern, so that deviations could be investigated at subsequent checking calls.

2.3 *Record keeping* Following the interview, children and their parents were shown how to use the scale and fill in the three different dietary record books. The pink A4 diary was to be kept at home and used for all other recording where proper weighing was possible. The A7 yellow pocket notebook, which was issued with a small pencil, was designed for children to carry around with them. It enabled them to record items which were brought and consumed away from home or school when weighing of foods was not possible, such as a bag of chips bought and consumed on the way home from school. Prices and descriptions were recorded.

2.4 *Record instructions* Fieldworkers stressed that all recording had to be clear and detailed because there would be follow-up questions on many items. Everything consumed was to be recorded, and for items recorded in the yellow pocket diary the price and place of purchase was to be recorded. Although water has no nutritional value, children were asked to record it because exceptions to rules can be confusing and only by recording all drinks can a coverage check be made on fluid consumption at the end of each day.

2.5 *Plate weights and zeroing* Children were shown how to zero the scales after each weighing so that a series of items put onto the same plate could be separately weighed. When really heavy plates were used the scale could overload, and in households which used such plates, the children were issued with a lightweight plastic plate to use instead.

2.6 *Practice session* Fieldworkers encouraged children to do some practice weighing with real food or drink and the procedure for weighing leftovers was demonstrated. This involved reweighing the original plate, now containing the leftovers and recording this weight, together with a tick next to all foods leftover, in the relevant column of the record book. The last meal was recalled in detail to give the child some practice in detailed recording and the importance of recording the bought form (eg tinned, fresh etc) and cooking methods was explained. Then, having answered any remaining questions from parents of children, the interviewer told the child to start full recording from that moment on and arranged to recall at the same time the next day. In fact, the first evening of recorded data was used to give the child practice in recording, and the analysis has been based on a 7 day record starting from the midnight which ended the placing day.

2.7 *The Checking Calls* The 24 hour checking call provided the first opportunity for the interviewer to assess how well the children understood the task required of them. Given the complexity of the records, an early 24 hour recall was essential so that any misunderstanding could be quickly made good, and interviewers were instructed to make this mandatory. The checking call procedure covered:

the individual food entries including

— time of consumption
— source of food
— adequacy of description
— the weight served
— presence of leftovers

and the food entries in context including

— whether recognisable meals were eaten each day

— whether the recorded pattern of eating was significantly different from the child's interview answers

— whether drinks had been recorded

— whether there was any record of snacks between meals.

2.8 *Methods of checking*

2.8.1 The fieldworker checked the food item recorded in detail using code lists and a checking aide-memoire card which listed details of all the types of food. Weights were scrutinised for feasibility. This identified where the scale had been misread, and where digits had been transposed in copying and where the scale had not been reset to zero between weighings. It detected those children who had weighed a common item once, such as the milk in a cup of tea and had simply copied the same weight on other occasions instead of weighing separately each time.

2.8.2 The interviewer asked probe questions to elicit missing information, but the checking call always ended with words of praise to the child for the recording done so far, encouragement for the future, and an appointment for the next checking call. The number of checking calls during the 7 day recording period varied from child to child; some children needed a call every day to keep recording up to scratch, but no child received fewer than 3 checking calls.

2.8.3 After each checking call the completed pages of the white diary were taken away by the interviewer and a note was made of unbranded purchased items recorded in the yellow notebook. The interviewer attempted to code all the foods recorded on these completed pages the following day. The nutritionist fieldwork advisers were telephoned about any queries and notes were made of any additional information required from probing questions at the next checking call. Fieldworkers were instructed to record full details of branded products but not to buy different locations. Instead branded products were purchased once from head office using the fieldworkers descriptions. The place of purchase for unbranded items in the yellow notebook items was visited to buy a duplicate item and check the description and weight of that item. With this additional information the yellow notebook items were transferred with full details onto the relevant day sheets of the white diary. Finally the number of meals, drinks, snacks and sweets was counted for each day in order to highlight "unusual" days which could have required extra checking questions.

2.8.4 At the final check call after the usual checks, there was a five minute closing interview about the 7 day period covering such topics as whether the child had been sick or away from school.

2.9 *Lunchtime observations* Apart from the home checking calls fieldworkers undertook direct monitoring of the children's record keeping through their school

254

observation calls. Interviewers called on the schools at lunchtime to observe and check that the sampled children were weighing all foods consumed and recording all leftovers. When watching the schoolmeal takers fieldworkers were instructed to note whether the survey children were being given larger portions of food than their peers. Only one such case was observed and that appeared to be a child who was regularly given larger helpings that his classmates—not just during the survey period. Otherwise, they were there to check that the children were recording in sufficient detail and to help any child whose slowness in weighing and recording was delaying proceedings in the school dining area. Children who brought, or were served, packed lunches at school were also monitored at these observation calls.

2.10   *Coding of the food and drink recorded*

2.10.1   *The food code list*   Each food had to be given a code number that would enable the computer to identify the energy and nutrient intake which it represented, though many foods had a variety of different codes to distinguish different cooking methods that would change the nutrient content, and there were a number of codes for prepared dishes. For each of these codes a nutrient content was available from one of five sources:

a.   "McCance and Widdowson's 'The Composition of Foods' " (Eds A A Paul and D A T Southgate), London: HMSO, 1978.

b.   The DHSS Food Composition Tables by M M Disselduff (unpublished).

c.   Wiles S, Nettleton P, Black A. Nutrient composition of some cooked dishes eaten in Britain: A supplementary food composition table. *Journal of Human Nutrition* 1980: *34*: 189.

d.   'Immigrant Foods'. Second Supplement to McCance and Widdowson's 'The Composition of Foods'. S P Tan, R W Wenlock and D H Buss. London: HMSO, 1985.

e.   'Cereals and Cereal Products'. Third Supplement to McCance and Widdowson's 'The Composition of Foods'. B Holland, I D Unwin and D H Buss. Letchworth: Royal Society of Chemistry, 1988.

Interviewers were not given the nutrient content of listed foods but they were issued with a food code list describing foods in sufficient detail to distinguish the required code numbers. The list which they were given contained about 1,080 different foods or food dishes.

2.10.2   *Coding the record book*   During training fieldworkers were taught to recognise the detail required to allocate the appropriate code number. The necessary detail was secured from the children at the time of the fieldwork while children or their mothers could still recall the precise nature of the items consumed. In cases where the recorded food was not on the list fieldworkers telephoned the nutritionist fieldwork advisers for guidance. Sometimes the recorded foods had to be 'split' into components which were codeable. So, for example, a cheese, ham and tomato pizza was split into cheese and tomato pizza, for which there was a code, and an entry of, say, 'tinned ham' for which there was also a code.

2.10.3   *Leftovers*   Food consumption surveys are more accurate when leftovers are properly weighed and deducted from the original served weights to yield net weights consumed. However, some people are apt to forget the weighing of leftovers no matter how diligent the interviewer may be in reminding them to do so. When making her checking call the interviewer can always probe for description of leftovers but there is no chance, at that stage, of securing the weight. Most commonly this problem arises when the subject neglects to weigh as leftovers the natural wastage of food item such as the bones in fish, the skin of a banana or the core of an apple. Food composition tables cope with this problem by the 'as purchased' codes which contain allowances for the non-edible part in the food composition analysis. Such codes are particularly useful but interviewers had to be trained to be especially careful that these 'as purchased' codes were only used in appropriate circumstance.

2.11 *Guidance from the nutritionist fieldwork advisers*

2.11.1 Inevitably the foods on the code list did not include every item eaten by the children. In all cases where the child's description did not match one of the foods described on the code list, interviewers were instructed to contact one of the fieldwork consultants at head office. Two nutritionists, Dr E Evans and Mrs A Melton, with considerable survey experience were available at head office to give advice in such cases. Sometimes this advice was that the food in questions was, in nutritional terms, such a close approximation to one of the foods which was on the code list that it could be split into its components and coded in that way, as explained above. On other occasions when further information about the food was needed, a recall on the child or the mother was recommended. If the nutritionist felt that the decision on coding required further thought, the entry was flagged for special attention when the completed diary reached head office.

2.11.2 Record books were scanned by the two nutritionists who would deal with the outstanding food coding queries and fill in weights for known sizes of branded goods. Following this, the record book and questionnaires were passed on for coding of time periods, social classes and other such tasks that could be undertaken by other staff. Before being passed for punching, record books were subjected to a final scrutiny by the nutritionist fieldwork advisers.

2.11.3 Nutritionist advisers made direct contact with all remote site kitchen supervisors to check details of school recipes or, in some cases where kitchen supervisors had already been seen by interviewers, in order to seek further clarification of some recipes.

Appendix C: Anthropometric Measurements

1. **Development of methodology**   The problems faced by the researchers were very
the thinking behind the methodology have been explained in some detail in the report
on that earlier research, (Knight I. *The Heights and Weights of Adults in Great Britain*,
London: HMSO, 1984) and they have not been reported in detail here.

2. **Weight measurement technique**   Children were weighed using a spring balance
with digital readout. The machine used was the SOEHNLE digital personal weighing
scale which has an electronic digital readout and is calibrated in units of 200g up to
135kg. These scales are self-zeroing, and they lock the readout once the child has
stayed on them for long enough to produce a stable measurement. Shoes and heavier
outer garments were removed prior to measurement, but although the child was asked
to indicate the clothing he/she was still wearing, no allowance has been made for the
weight of that clothing in the results which this report contains.

3. **Height measurement technique**   It is generally known that the erect height of a
person declines as the day progresses and the measurement of maximum height clearly
requires some stretch of the spine, as well as the correct general posture. Fieldworkers
were trained to explain the importance of posture including the need for the head to be
in the Frankfort Plane. Placing the head in the Frankfort Plane requires that the line
between the base of the ocular socket and the external auditory meatus is horizontal.
The requirement for stretch was fully explained to the fieldworkers and they were
taught to use the unsupported stretch system which had worked successfully in the
OPCS adult heights and weights survey.

4. **Field procedure**

4.1   Subjects were asked to remove their shoes and heavy outer garments.
Fieldworkers demonstrated the Frankfort Plane position to the household, and asked
the child to indicate what he/she was still wearing on a self completion form printed at
the back of the socio-economic questionnaire.

4.2   The equipment was set up, with scales on a hard flat surface.

4.3   The subject was positioned on the scales platform and asked to look straight
ahead, standing relaxed but still. The interviewer would then take a weight reading
from the digital readout.

4.4   The subject was then positioned on the stadiometer. All fieldworkers were
trained to follow a standard procedure:

a.   Check that subject's feet were together and heels against the back plate, flat on the board.

b.   Check that the subject's arms were held loosely by his/her side.

c.   Check Frankfort Plane position (using a straight edge).

d.   Ask the subject to stretch with the request "Now stand up as tall as you can." (Interviewers checked that a height increase occurred).

e.   Recheck the head position (Frankfort Plane), and heels before accepting the measurement.

In cases where the heel or Frankfort Plane positioning was lost or a height increase did not occur, the child was asked to relax, the stadiometer reset and the procedure repeated, with any faults in positioning corrected.

Appendix D: Forms used in the Survey

1. Record book for food eaten at school

2. Socio-economic questionnaire

3. Pocket book

4. Home record book

5. School questionnaire

S1187 SCHOOL CHILDRENS DIETARY SURVEY

Interviewer No.		▨

Area	Grp	Child

HOME RECORD BOOK

Please record all food and drink as
shown inside

First name ———————————

Office of Population Censuses and Surveys
Social Survey Division
St Catherines House
London
WC2B 6JP

HOW TO USE THIS BOOK

Remember to write down everything you eat or drink, whether at mealtimes or in between - even medicines should be included.

Please START EACH DAY ON A NEW SHEET - but you can use more than one sheet a day if necessary.

Remember to write down the day and date at the top of each sheet.

HOW TO WEIGH

Press button on scales to switch on and make green zero show.

Weigh container (plate, cup or bowl) and write the weight in column D.

Leave plate on scales and press button to set scale back to zero.

Write down description of first food in column C, put it on the plate and write weight in column D.

Leave plate on scales and set scale back to zero (press button).

Put second food on plate, write down description, and write weight down in column D.

Leave plate on scales and set scale back to zero.

Repeat for each item of food or drink.

NOW EAT IT!

Weight plate with any leftovers (if there are any) and tick to show which foods were leftover.

DESCRIBING FOOD AND DRINK

Column A: Choose the right number from the list at the top of the sheet to show where the food came from and write that number down in the first column.

Column B: Write down the time when food or drink was eaten.

Column C: Put down the description of food, EACH ITEM ON A SEPARATE LINE. Please give as much information as possible - type of food, name, and how it was cooked.

Column D: Write in the weight of the food or drink.

Column E: Write down the weight of the plate with left-overs on it and tick which items were left over.

After everything on your plate is written down, leave a line blank before your next plate.

(i)

Whenever you weight anything always start with a plate, bowl or cup, please never put food directly onto the scales.

For foods that already come in containers like yogurt or trifles you can weigh the unopened container and then weigh the container again when you have eaten the food. Or if you prefer you can tip out the food into a bowl which you have just weighed.

To weigh bread and butter or anything else you spread on bread, start by weighing the plate as usual. Press the button again to set scale back to zero and weigh the bread. Press the button again to set the scale back to zero then remove the bread and quickly spread the butter on. Put the bread back on the scales and it will show the weight of the butter or margarine you have just put on. Now set the scale back to zero and then remove the bread again to quickly spread the jam or marmite. Put the bread back on the scale and it will show the weight of the jam you have put on.

If there are any leftovers we need to know about them. You should weight the plate with the leftovers on it and put the weight in column E next to the weight you wrote down for the empty plate.   Then be sure to put a tick next to each type of food that was left over.

If something was spilt write into the leftovers column about how much you think was lost; for example "about ½ spilt".

If you are eating somewhere that you cannot weight the food, then write down the most information you can in your yellow pocket notebook. For example a meal in a cafe like this:

| 12·30 | In the Broadway Cafe
Bacon sandwich in white bread
(full round) Cost   40p
Large mug of coffee   20p
Apple pie   25p | left ¼ |

or a mars bar on the way home, like this;

| 4·05 | Mars bar 16p | |

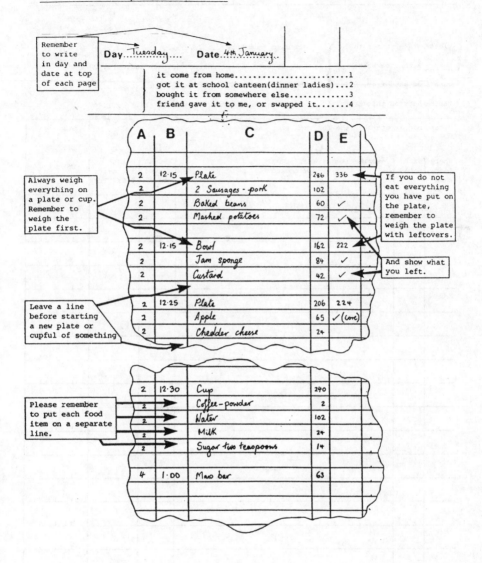

Remember to write in day and date at top of each page

Day Tuesday.... **Date** 4th January..

it come from home...........................1
got it at school canteen(dinner ladies)...2
bought it from somewhere else.............3
friend gave it to me, or swapped it.......4

A	B	C	D	E
2	12·15	Plate	286	336
2		2 Sausages - pork	102	
2		Baked beans	60	✓
2		Mashed potatoes	72	✓
2	12·15	Bowl	162	222
2		Jam sponge	84	✓
2		Custard	42	✓
2	12·25	Plate	206	224
2		Apple	65	✓ (core)
2		Cheddar cheese	24	
2	12·30	Cup	240	
2		Coffee-powder	2	
2		Water	102	
2		Milk	24	
2		Sugar two teaspoons	14	
4	1·00	Mars bar	63	

Always weigh everything on a plate or cup. Remember to weigh the plate first.

Leave a line before starting a new plate or cupful of something

Please remember to put each food item on a separate line.

If you do not eat everything you have put on the plate, remember to weigh the plate with leftovers.

And show what you left.

Day .... Date .... | Day Order...... |

write in
col. A

Please write number in ⎫   it came from home 1

column A to show where   got it from school canteen (dinner ladies).. 2

each food came from, using ⎬   bought it from somewhere else 3

the numbers on this list. ⎭   friend gave it to me, or swapped it 4

Please use a separate line for each item eaten.

A	B	C	D	E	FOR OFFICE USE ONLY
Where food came from	Time eaten	Describe item – What it was – How cooked	Weight served grms.	Weight of leftovers TICK ITEMS	

pink

264

	Area No.		School	Serial no.	

Post code of home [   ]

Interviewer number [▨]

Date of interview [8 3]

Details of selected child

First Name		Sex		Age group		Date of birth			A C W
1		M F	10/11	14/15					
		1 2	1	2					1 2 3

List other household members in relationship to selected child

	Relationship to sampled CHILD	OFF USE	AGE Parents and children ONLY	COMMON CATERING		MARITAL STATUS			EMPLOYMENT			Age of leaving f/t education	A C W N
				Yes	No	Mar.	Sin.	W/D/S	P/t.	F/t	None		
2	Mother			1	2	1	2	3	1	2	3		1 2 3 4
3	Father			1	2	1	2	3	1	2	3		1 2 3 4
4				1	2								
5				1	2								
6				1	2								
7				1	2								
8				1	2								
9				1	2								
10				1	2								
11				1	2								

TO MARRIED WOMEN WITH NO HUSBAND IN HOUSEHOLD - Others go to next page

8 Is your husband absent because he usually works away from home, or for some other reason ?

Usually works away 1

INCL. ARMED FORCES & MERCHANT NAVY

Some other reason 2

— go to Q9

1

265

| | | 1 | CODE 1 FOR OFFICE USE (IPF) |

IF "FATHER" IS WORKING ASK OF HIM:

DNA No father living there ...	2	go to Q11
DNA Father not working	3	go to Q10

9 And can I just check what is your/your partner's job? What do you/does he actually do?

PROBE

FULLY

go to Q11

on page 3

Employee	1
Self employed	2

IF FATHER NOT WORKING

10 Are you .... PROBE AND CODE ONE ONLY

out of employment but seeking work	1	
out of employment because of sickness or injury but intending to seek work	2	
sick or injured but NOT intending to seek work	3	ask (a) and (b)
None of these .... SPECIFY	4	go to Q11

(a) How many weeks have you/has he been away from work?

RECORD ⟶ ----- ASK (b)

(b) What was your/his job when last in employment?

OCCUPATION

go to Q11

Employee 1	
Self-employed 2	

Yellow   2

11 Does .... (CHILD) ever have
    school dinners during term time?

Yes	1	ask (a)
No	2	go to Q12

    IF YES
    (a) On how many days each week
        does .... (CHILD) usually have
        school dinners?

        RECORD NO. OF DAYS ─────────────▶

12 What did .... (CHILD) do for his/her
    mid-day meal most days of last
    (school) week?

Had school dinner	1
Took packed lunch	2
Came home for lunch	3
Went to home of relative or friend	4
Went to cafe/take away	5
Bought food on the way to school .	6
Other (SPECIFY)	
Does not have mid-day meal	9

13 Does .... (CHILD) have milk at
    school?

Yes	1	- ask (a)
No	2	- see Q14

    IF YES
    (a) How much do you pay for
        the milk?

Does not pay (free) ...	1	see Q4
Pays this amount ──────▶		
		pence
Period: each day	1	⎫ see Q14
each week ...	2	⎭

Others . |..DNA..| - see Q15

14 Do you have to pay for school
dinners or do you get them free?

Pays for school dinners	1	ask (i)
Gets them free	2	go to (ii)

IF PAYS
(i) Does .... (CHILD) take money when
(s)he stays to school dinner and
choose what (s)he wants to buy
from the school canteen, or is
the school meal provided for a
fixed price?

Chooses what (s)he wants to buy..	1	go to (a)
Fixed price meal	2	go to (b)

IF GETS DINNERS FREE
(ii) Do you give .... (CHILD) any
money to spend at the school
canteen?

Yes	1	ask (a)
No	2	see Q15

(a) How much did you give
him/her to spend today
at the school canteen?

RECORD ⟶ | | see Q15

(b) What is the price of
a school meal at his/
her school?

RECORD ⟶

IF CHILD BUYS FOOD ON WAY TO SCHOOL/AT CAFE (Q12)

Others .... | DNA | go to Q16

15 You mentioned that .... (CHILD) buys something
out to eat at mid-day. How much did you give
him/her today to spend on his/her mid-day meal?

RECORD AMOUNT IN PENCE ⟶ | | P
(record 99p or over as 99)

4

268

16 Are there any foods which .... (CHILD) doesn't
    eat because (s)he doesn't like them?

        IF YES: SPECIFY   Yes   1

                                                No   2

17 Are there any particular foods which .... (CHILD)
    does not eat for health or other reasons

                                                Yes   1   SPECIFY

                                                No   2   go to Q1

Food type	Reason

18 Does .... (CHILD) usually take
    sugar in tea or coffee?

                        Yes, sugar in tea   1
                        Yes, sugar in coffee   2
                        No, sugar in neither tea nor coffee   3
                        Does not drink tea or coffee   4

19 Does .... (CHILD) usually have a
    breakfast before he/she goes to
    school, or doesn't he/she bother?

                                Usually has breakfast .   1
                                Doesn't bother   2

5

269

20 What about Saturdays and Sundays;
    does .... (CHILD) usually have
    breakfast at weekends or doesn't
    he/she bother?

                          Usually has breakfast .   1

                          Doesn't bother   2

21 When you cook mincemeat or stews, do
    you skim the fat off the top before serving
    the food out, or does your family prefer
    the fat left in the food?

                          skims fat off   1

                          prefer fat left in food ...   2

22 When you make gravy, do you add
    thickening or additional flavouring?

        PROMPT   adds thickening............   1

          AS   adds additional flavouring.   2

        NECESSARY   adds both   3

                          Neither   4

23 When you buy bread for the family
    do you always buy one kind of
    bread, or do you buy more than
    one kind of bread?

                          always buy one kind   1

                          buys more than one kind   2

    (a) Which kind(s) of bread do you buy?

                              White   1

             CODE   Hovis   2

             ALL   Wholemeal   3

             THAT   Slimcea/Procea   4

             APPLY   Other (SPECIFY).......   5

24 What kind of milk do you have?

    (a) Any other kinds?

6

270

25 Now thinking back to when .... (CHILD) was born.
Can you remember, was he/she born
earlier than expected?

Yes	1	ask (a)
No not earlier	2	go to Q26-28
(Volunteered) Not natural mother ...	3	see Q29
only		

IF YES
(a) How many weeks early?

CODE TO NEAREST WHOLE WEEK ───┤- - - - - -

26 How much did (s)he weigh
at birth?

Pounds   ounces

27 Where was .... (CHILD) born, I mean
in which town and country?

RECORD (NEAREST) TOWN BELOW, WITH COUNTRY.
RECORD COUNTRY IF ABROAD

28 Can I just check then, how many children
have you had, I mean all those who are
living now (no matter what age) plus any
who have died but survived until the age
of 5 including .... (CHILD)?

RECORD NUMBER ─────────────►- - - - - -

IF MORE THAN ONE

DNA Only one child ....X ────────► go to Q32
(a) Is .... (CHILD) your eldest child,
or the second (or which)?

RECORD BIRTH ORDER ─────────►- - - - - -

7

271

IF INTENDING TO MEASURE AT SCHOOL

DNA will measure child at home .... go to Q30 with
preamble about
measuring child

29 Part of this survey is to measure the
height and weight of all children in
the sample. May we measure .... (CHILD)'s
height and weight at school?

Yes 1   ask Q30

No 2   go to Q31

30 We often find that there is a link
between a child's height and weight
and the height of his natural parents.
Are you (and your husband) the
natural parents of .... (CHILD)?

Yes both are natural parents 1

only Mother is natural 2   see below

only Father is natural 3

neither are natural parents 4   see Q31

ASK FOR NATURAL PARENTS:

	Feet	inches
Father's height ———▶		

	Feet	inches
Mother's height ———▶		

	Stones	pounds
Father's weight ———▶		

	Stones	pounds
Mother's weight ———▶		

8

DNA Mother not employed/no mother ....x ──────────► go to Q36

31 You told me earlier that you have a job.
    Can you tell me what your (main) job is?
    What do you actually do?

                                    Employee........ 1

                                    Self employed .. 2

32 On which days of the week do you
    usually work?

                        Monday 1

            CODE   Tuesday 1
            ALL
            THAT   Wednesday 1
            APPLY
                        Thursday 1

                        Friday 1

                        Saturday 1

                        Sunday 1

            (SPON) No usual pattern of Work 1

33. How many hours a week do you
    usually work leaving out meal breaks?

                RECORD TO NEAREST HOUR ──────────► ------

34 What time do you usually leave
    home to go to work?

                    Does paid work at home 1
                                                        ┐ go to Q36
                    No usual time, varies a lot. 2   ┘

        RECORD TIME IF GIVEN (24hr Clock) ──►

35 And what time do you usually
    get home from work?

            RECORD TIME (24hr Clock) ──────►

9

273

36 Can you look at this card and tell
    me which group covers the total
    NET income (of you and your spouse) usually have
    from all sources: that is after deduction
    of tax and national insurance, but
    including any pensions or benefits?

	Weekly		Monthly	
A	£30 or less	£130 or less	A	1
B	Over £30 – 40	Over £130 – 173	B	2
C	Over £40 – 50	Over £173 – 217	C	3
D	Over £50 – 60	Over £217 – 260	D	4
E	Over £60 – 80	Over £260 – 347	E	5
F	Over £80 – 100	Over £347 – 433	F	6
G	Over £100 – 125	Over £433 – 542	G	7
H	Over £125 – 150	Over £542 – 650	H	8
J	Over £150	Over £650	J	9

37 Can I just check are you currently receiving
    Family Income Supplement (FIS)?

    Yes 1
    No 2

38 And have you or your husband drawn
    Supplementary Benefit at any time
    in the last 14 days?

    Yes 1
    No 2

10

274

39 Now can you tell me what you usually have to eat and drink in a day,
    starting with when you get up and going right through the day to the time
    you go to bed? RECORD APPROXIMATE TIMES, FOOD DESCRIPTIONS.

In bed or before breakfast

Breakfast

During the morning

Mid-day

During the afternoon

When you get home from school

During the evening

Before going to bed/in bed

11

275

DNA Others ──────────────────→ go to Q41

40 On school days, what time do you
    usually eat your main meal at school?

    RECORD (24hr CLOCK) ────→

41 What time do you leave for school in
    the morning?

                                    hr │ mins

    RECORD ──────────────────→

42 Do you ever buy sweets or snacks to
    eat on the way to, or back from, school?

                        Yes 1

                        No 2

43 When you are at school, do you ever buy sweets,
    crisps or drinks at breaktime?

                        Yes 1

                        No 2

END OF
PLACEMENT
SCHEDULE

12

TO INTERVIEWER

A Does school offer a fixed price meal
   and cafeteria choice as well?

Yes, both .... Y

No .... N

B Did child have any school dinners
   during the recording week?

Yes .... Y

No .... N

TO CHILD

IF YES TO BOTH A and B ABOVE - others go to Q2

1. Did you choose the fixed price meal at school
    on any of your record keeping days?

No .... N

IF YES
(a) On which days?

Monday	1	IF ALL 5
Tuesday	2	DAYS CODED
Wednesday	3	GO TO Q3
Thursday	4	OTHERWISE
Friday	5	ASK Q2

CODE ALL

THAT APPLY

2. And thinking back over the past 7 days
    did you go to a cafe or take-away for
    your midday meal?

Yes	1	ask (b)
No	2	ask (a)

(a) Again in the last 7 days, did you buy
    all, or most, of the food for your
    midday meal on the way to school?

Yes	1
No	2

(b) On which days
    (FOR EITHER 2 or (a) ABOVE)

Monday	1
Tuesday	2
Wednesday	3
Thursday	4
Friday	5

3. Have you been unwell at any time
    in the past 7 days?

Yes	1	go to Q4
No	2	SPECIFY ILLNESS AND DAYS THEN ASK Q4

13

277

4. Have you been away from school on any
   day in the past 7 days?

   Yes 1   ask (a)
   No 2   go to Q5

   IF YES
   (a) On how many school days, in the
       last 7 days, were you off school?

                    RECORD NO. OF DAYS

5. Have you been to any parties or had any
   special meals in the past 7 days?

   Yes 1
   No 2

6. Are there any other unusual circumstances
   which may have affected your eating
   habits during the last 7 days?

   Yes 1   SPECIFY, THEN
   No 2   DEAL WITH
                       HEIGHT AND
                       WEIGHT

278

INTERVIEWER NOTE OF ANY SPECIAL CIRCUMSTANCES

Childs height [| | . |] centimetres

Posture	1
Hat/Turban	2
Carpet	3

Weight [| | |] kilos

BOYS CLOTHES	
ITEMS WORN WHILST BEING WEIGHED	
Pair of socks	01
Pants/briefs	02
Vest	03
T Shirt	04
Shirt	05
Trousers/jeans	06
Kilt	07
Belt/braces	08
Jumper	09
Cardigan	10
Tie/cravat	11
Something else not on list (SPECIFY)	

GIRLS CLOTHES	
ITEMS WORN WHILST BEING WEIGHED	
Pair of socks	01
Stockings/Tights	02
Suspender Belt	03
Pants/Briefs	04
Corset/Girdle	05
Bra	06
Slip/Underskirt	07
Vest	08
Blouse	09
T-Shirt	10
Skirt	11
Trousers	12
Belt	13
Dress	14
Jumper	15
Cardigan	16
Waistcoat/Jerkin	17
Something else not on list (SPECIFY)	

OFFICE USE

	School meal	Went home for lunch or to friend/relative	Cafe/takeaway, or on way to school	Other
Monday	1	2	3	4
Tuesday	1	2	3	4
Wednesday	1	2	3	4
Thursday	1	2	3	4
Friday	1	2	3	4

16   W2425A OPCS 11/82

280

Pocket Book

Please use this notebook to write down any food or drink you have away from home or school

S1187
OPCS
St Catherines House
10 Kingsway
London WC2

Day................. Date.................

Time eaten	Description (please include price, who made it and where it was bought)	Any leftovers?

CONFIDENTIAL

S1187 SCHOOL CHILDRENS DIETARY SURVEY

			▨

Interviewer No.

Area | Grp | Child

HOME RECORD BOOK

Please record all food and drink as
shown inside

First name ——————————————

The interviewer will call again:

Day	Date	Time

Office of Population Censuses and Surveys
Social Survey Division
St Catherines House
London
WC2B 6JP

282

Remember to write down everything you eat or drink, whether at mealtimes or in between - even medicines should be included.

Please START EACH DAY ON A NEW SHEET - but you can use more than one sheet a day if necessary.

Remember to write down the day and date at the top of each sheet.

HOW TO WEIGH

Press button on scales to switch on and make green zero show.

Weigh container (plate, cup or bowl) and write the weight in column D.

Leave plate on scales and press button to set scale back to zero.

Write down description of first food in column C, put it on the plate and write weight in column D.

Leave plate on scales and set scale back to zero (press button).

Put second food on plate, write down description, and write weight down in column D.

Leave plate on scales and set scale back to zero.

Repeat for each item of food or drink.

NOW EAT IT!

Weight plate with any leftovers (if there are any) and tick to show which foods were leftover.

DESCRIBING FOOD AND DRINK

Column B: Write down the time when food or drink was eaten.

Column C: Put down the description of food, EACH ITEM ON A SEPARATE LINE. Please give as much information as possible - type of food, name, and how it was cooked.

Column D: Write in the weight of the food or drink.

Column E: Write down the weight of the plate with left-overs on it and tick which items were left over.

After everything on your plate is written down, leave a line blank before your next plate.

(i)

Whenever you weight anything always start with a plate, bowl or cup, please never put food directly onto the scales.

For foods that already come in containers like yogurt or trifles you can weigh the unopened container and then weigh the container again when you have eaten the food. Or if you prefer you can tip out the food into a bowl which you have just weighed.

To weigh bread and butter or anything else you spread on bread, start by weighing the plate as usual. Press the button again to set scale back to zero and weigh the bread. Press the button again to set the scale back to zero then remove the bread and quickly spread the butter on. Put the bread back on the scales and it will show the weight of the butter or margarine you have just put on. Now set the scale back to zero and then remove the bread again to quickly spread the jam or marmite. Put the bread back on the scale and it will show the weight of the jam you have put on.

If there are any leftovers we need to know about them. You should weight the plate with the leftovers on it and put the weight in column E next to the weight you wrote down for the empty plate. Then be sure to put a tick next to each type of food that was left over.

If something was spilt write into the leftovers column about how much you think was lost; for example "about ½ spilt".

If you are eating somewhere that you cannot weight the food, then write down the most information you can in your yellow pocket notebook. For example a meal in a cafe like this:

| 12·30 | In the Broadway Cafe Bacon sandwich in white bread (full round) Cost 40p Large mug of coffee 20p Apple pie 25p | left ½ |

or a mars bar on the way home, like this;

| 4·05 | Mars bar 16p | |

(ii)

284

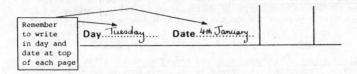

Remember to write in day and date at top of each page

Day Tuesday..... Date 4th January..

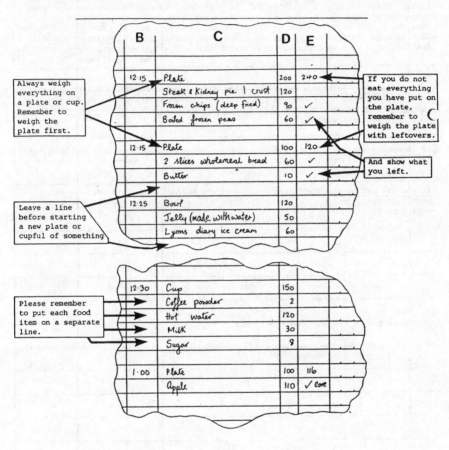

Always weigh everything on a plate or cup. Remember to weigh the plate first.

If you do not eat everything you have put on the plate, remember to weigh the plate with leftovers.

And show what you left.

Leave a line before starting a new plate or cupful of something

Please remember to put each food item on a separate line.

	B	C	D	E
	12·15	Plate	200	240
		Steak & Kidney pie 1 crust	120	
		Frozen chips (deep fried)	90	✓
		Boiled frozen peas	60	✓
	12·15	Plate	100	120
		2 slices wholemeal bread	60	✓
		Butter	10	✓
	12·25	Bowl	120	
		Jelly (made with water)	50	
		Lyons diary ice cream	60	
	12·30	Cup	150	
		Coffee powder	2	
		Hot water	120	
		Milk	30	
		Sugar	9	
	1·00	Plate	100	116
		Apple	110	✓ core

Day .... Date .... | Day order .....

Did you have a school dinner today?   Yes [ ] Please

                                       No [ ] tick

Please use a separate line for each item eaten

B	C	D	E	FOR OFFICE USE ONLY

Time eaten	Describe item - Brand
	         - Fresh/frozen/dried etc
	         - How cooked
		Weight served grms.	Weight of leftovers TICK ITEMS	

White

286

School Children's Dietary Survey S1187

<table>
<tr><td></td></tr>
<tr><td>School Number</td></tr>
</table>

<table>
<tr><td></td><td></td></tr>
<tr><td colspan="2">interviewer nos.</td></tr>
</table>

School Questionnaire

School name _____

Office of Population Censuses and Surveys
St Catherines House
10 Kingsway
London
WC2B 6JP

287

ASK OF NOMINATED CONTACT OR SCHOOL SECRETARY

1. Does the school have a tuck shop or similar
   arrangement within the school grounds, but
   <u>independent</u> of the school meals service?

	Yes	1	ask (a)
	No	2	go to Q2

   IF YES
   (a) Do the staff run this "tuck shop" or
   is it run by the children/parents?

run by teaching staff	1
run by children/parents	2
run by children under staff supervision	3

   (b) During which hours is the
   "tuck shop" open?

   RECORD

   (d) And does the "tuck shop" sell ...

	YES	NO
Milk?	1	2
Tea/coffee?	1	2
Soft drinks?	1	2
Sweets or biscuits?.	1	2
Crisps?	1	2
Sandwiches?	1	2

   INDIVIDUAL PROMPT

   any other type of food?—
   IF YES SPECIFY ◄

288

2. Does the school have vending machines
   within the school grounds for use by
   the children?

   Yes .... 1 | ask (a)

   No .... 2 | go to Q3

   IF YES
   (a) Do the 10/14 year olds have
       access to them?

   Yes .... 1 | ask (i)

   No .... 2 | go to Q3

   IF YES
   (i) During which hours are the
       children allowed to use the
       vending machines?

           RECORD

   (ii) Do the machines sell ......

	YES	NO
Milk?	1	2
Tea/coffee?	1	2
Soft drinks?	1	2
Sweets or biscuits?	1	2
Crisps?	1	2
Sandwiches?	1	2

INDIVIDUAL
PROMPT

3. Is the school meals service responsible
   for the vending machines in this school?

   Yes 1

   No 2

4. Is there a shop or cafe or
   take-away very near to
   the school?

                                            Yes 1   ask (a)
                                            No 2   go to Q5

   IF YES
   (a) Can the 10/14 year olds
       use it at lunchtime?

                              Yes they all can 1

                              Yes if they don't
                                stay to school dinners 2

                              No 3

5. Do hot dog vans, ice cream vans or
   any other such vans wait outside
   the school?

                                            Yes 1   ask (a)
                                            No 2   see 6

   IF YES
   (a) At what times?

6. INTERVIEWER CHECK
   Does the school meals service
   provide school dinners at this
   school for all children who want them
   or only those entitled to free meals?

                         for all who want them 1   ask sections
                                                                 B and C

                         for "free meals" children only ... 2   ask section B

                         No school dinners provided 3   make notes

290

TO KITCHEN/DINING ROOM SUPERVISOR

7. Does the school meals service offer
   hot food at this school?

Yes	1	go to Q8
No	2	ask (a)

   IF NO
(a) Do you serve sandwiches, rolls
    and snacks only, or do you
    also serve other foods?

Only sandwiches, rolls and snacks.....	1
Other foods	2

   IF OTHER FOODS: SPECIFY TYPES OF OTHER FOOD SERVED

8. Is the food prepared at the school
   or is it prepared elsewhere?

Prepared here ...	1	ask (i)
Elsewhere	2	go to Q9

   IF PREPARED HERE
   (i) Do you use the traditional
       recipe book in the
       preparation of meals here?

Yes	1
No	2

   (ii) Do you add extra dried skimmed milk
        to recipes as was recommended in
        the traditional recipe book?

Yes	1	ask (iii)
No	2	see Q10

   IF YES
   (iii) Do you add it to...

INDIVIDUAL PROMPT	School custard?	1	
	Mashed potato?	1	see Q10
	White sauces?	1	
	or other main courses like stews?	1	

   IF FOOD NOT PREPARED HERE
9. Where is the food prepared?

   RECORD ADDRESS AND (IF KNOWN)

   NAME OF KITCHEN SUPERVISOR

   WHERE FOOD IS PREPARED

Section C (Ask ONLY if school meals are available to all children)

TO THE KITCHEN/DINING ROOM SUPERVISOR

10. Does the school meals service at this school
    offer a cash cafeteria? I mean a choice of
    foods individually priced and available
    in any combination.

Yes	1	ask (a)
No	2	go to Q11

IF YES
(a) Do the children receiving free school
    meals "pay" with a fixed value token?

Yes, fixed value token	1	ask (b)
No, other means	2	go to Q11

IF YES
(b) What is the value of the token?

RECORD ———————▶		pence

11. Does the school meals service here (also)
    offer a menu (at least 2 courses) for
    a fixed price?

Yes	1	ask (a)
No	2	GO TO Q12

(a) What is the fixed price

RECORD ———————▶		pence
price varies	01	go to Q12

12. Do you offer a mixed price main dish each
    day? I mean a priced plate with a main
    item and associated vegetable?

Yes	1
No	2

IF YES
(a) Does this apply only to salads?

Yes	1
No	2

(b) What is the fixed price?

RECORD ———————▶		go to Q13
price varies	01	

13. Does the school meals service sell food to
    the children at any time before 11.30 in
    the morning or after 2.30 in the afternoon?

Yes	1
No	2

    IF YES: SPECIFY WHAT IS SERVED AND WHEN

292

PAYING FOR MEALS

14. Do the children buy meal tickets or pay for
    their meals before they enter the dining hall?

Yes	1
No	2

IF YES
(a) Do they pay or buy their tickets ......

daily, ...	1
once a week	2
or over a longer period?	3

SPECIFY ⌐
←

Remainder: Arrange to check recipe content of any school meals
your sampled children consume, when you have finished with that school.

Printed in the United Kingdom for Her Majesty's Stationery Office.
Dd.291384, 5/89, C35, 3385/4, 5673, 56884.